The Only Cure for Constipation

What Everyone Should Know About Constipation

S. H. Shepherd

The Only Cure for Constipation

The Only Cure for Constipation. Copyright © 2023. All rights reserved.

This book is for reference and informational purposes only and is in no way intended as medical counseling or medical advice. The author and publisher shall have neither liability nor responsibility to any person or entity with respect to any loss, damage, or injury caused or alleged to be caused directly or indirectly by the information contained in this book. If medical advice is required, the services of a competent professional should be sought.

No part of this book may be used or reproduced in any manner whatsoever without written permission except in cases of brief quotations (less than three hundred words) embodied in critical articles and reviews.

Scripture verses are mainly taken from the NKJV of the Holy Bible.

Cover design: Ljiljana Smilevski.

Contents

Prologue 4
Preface 6
Chapter 1   The Digestive System 7
Chapter 2   The American/Western Diet 13
Chapter 3   Common GI Problems 15
Chapter 4   Standard Treatments for Constipation 40
Chapter 5   Aging and Constipation 57
Chapter 6   Alcohol and Constipation 61
Chapter 7   Nocturia and Constipation 62
Chapter 8   Proper Food Combinations 63
Chapter 9   The Best Medicine 71
Chapter 10 Detoxification 80
Chapter 11 The Causes of Disease 86
Chapter 12 The Cure for Constipation 114
Chapter 13 Becoming Your Own Doctor 120
Chapter 14 Dangers to Avoid 127
Chapter 15 Abiding by Nature's Laws 142
Chapter 16 Obesity 145
Chapter 17 Colonics and Enemas 149
Chapter 18 What Everyone Should Know About Fiber 153
Chapter 19 The Blood 162
Chapter 20 Antioxidants 168
Chapter 21 The Foods We Should Eat and Why 173
Chapter 22 The Food Pyramid 192
Chapter 23 How Eating Habits Are Formed 197
Chapter 24 Sleep and Constipation 201
Next Steps 206
About the Author 207
Bibliography 208
Appendices 213
Index 228

Prologue

Constipation is a disease that everyone seems to have but no one seems to know how to cure. It is known as an "idiopathic" disease in the medical literature, meaning that its cause is unknown, and this is evidenced by how mainstream medicine views constipation – as an affliction to be treated by medication (drugs). Drugs may temporarily alleviate the symptoms, but they can worsen the condition and more importantly they cannot cure constipation because drugs do not possess the ability to cure.

Constipation is the most prevalent gastrointestinal problem in the Western world.[1] It is estimated that very few people live without it. It is experienced by so many people that it is considered a normal part of life. It is perhaps the most common sign of ill health in people, even more so than the common cold. But unlike the common cold, it does not go away on its own. It is a dysfunction, an abnormality, a sign that something is wrong with the body.

It can be life-threatening, because if left uncorrected it can cause many life-shortening diseases because of its internal poisoning, typically organ and blood poisoning, that occurs when the body becomes imbued with toxins because of the blocked intestinal wastes. It can increase the risk of colon cancer, stomach cancer and pancreatic cancer, and can lead to nervous disorders, kidney disease and heart attacks.

Since what affects one part of the body affects all parts in some way, constipation can cause or contribute to heart disease, kidney disease and brain disease,[2][3] which are the first, second and sixth

---

[1] https://gi.org/topics/constipation-and-defection-problems/.
[2] https://www.ncbi.nlm.nih.gov/pmc/articles/PMC6399019/.

The Only Cure for Constipation

leading causes of death in the US.[4] Were these things widely known, constipation would not be considered just an ordinary health risk as many believe it is, but a risk to life itself.

I am convinced after devoting 30 years of life in the human health field and putting into practice what I learned to cure myself and others of constipation, that everyone should learn about this most troublesome and dangerous disease, and a disease it surely is for it was not meant that we should have it; and that, by learning about it, be able to cure themselves of it and live a healthy and vibrant life.

This book describes how to be constipation-free. It presents facts, not myths, about this medically ill-understood disease. It makes sense out of the mystery and doubt that surrounds the subject. It speaks frankly and honestly about its causes, its symptoms and its cure.

It discusses the standard medical treatments typically used, and describes their side effects. It explains why modern medicine cannot cure the disease.

It reveals how practically anyone can end that nagging feeling that something is not right about their health, and start living a constipation-free life, one that is fully in accord with how God intended for us to live. It explains what foods are the real culprits and why. It is not about using drugs or other palliative measures that do not cure, but about how constipation is cured using commonsense and old school wisdom.

---

[3] https://www.hopkinsmedicine.org/health/wellness-and-prevention/gastrointestinal-issues-whats-your-brain-have-to-do-with-it.
[4] https://www.medicalnewstoday.com/articles/282929#stroke-and-cerebrovascular-diseases.

Preface

I had constipation most of my life, not knowing why. I thought irregularity was a normal, natural part of living, and it was why they made laxatives. My parents never told me any different, nor did anyone else, as is the case with most people. But when I found out that being constipated was actually abnormal and a sign of ill health, a sign that something is wrong with the body, I set about how it may best be cured.

It is only natural that the body should want to freely expel what it freely ingests. But in today's culture with its emphasis on eating animal-based foods and fats and oils, it is not able to do so because these foods clog up the system and prolong the transit times of the wastes.

Those who wish to be cured of this "idiopathic" disease and live a genuine healthy life, should understand its causes, for disease cannot be cured without attacking its underlying causes. The best time to learn about constipation is now, not later in life, not when or if the time ever comes, which it never does, for you may never know if you do not know now.

The solution to constipation is not found in mainstream medicine. Research has shown that constipation, like with many other sicknesses and diseases, comes about almost invariably because of the foods that people eat. In fact, it is the major and often the only cause. It is not recognized as such by mainstream medicine primarily because medical professionals for the most part eat the same foods as almost everyone else.

The only "medicine" recommended in this book is that proved to have its marvelous effects on thousands of people.

Chapter 1 The Digestive System

The human organism as designed by God is about as perfect as anything can possibly be. It is what we do with it and put into it that makes the body less than perfect, and, apart from old age, it is the main reason we have sicknesses and diseases. The cure for constipation begins with a basic understanding of this fact. it is supplemented by a basic understanding of how the body digests food.

Digestion is a complex process that basically includes: 1) mechanical digestion (or chewing), and 2) chemical digestion and absorption.[5]

The digestive system is called the gastrointestinal (GI) tract, which is the 30-foot or so long series of hollow organs that move ingested food and liquids through the body and help digest them. They include: the mouth, which provides saliva and teeth for chewing, the esophagus that connects the mouth and the stomach, the stomach, which does a lot of the digesting, the pancreas, which supplies hormones and enzymes to breakdown the food, the small intestine, which continues digestion and absorbs nutrients into the bloodstream, and the large intestine, which completes the nutrient absorption and turns undigested food into stool.[6]

Most of the length of the GI tract is taken up by the intestines, with the small intestine being about 10-16 feet long and the large intes-

---

[5] https://guides.hostos.cuny.edu/bio140/5-16.
[6] https://www.niddk.nih.gov/health-information/digestive-diseases/digestive-system-how-it-works#:~:text=The%20digestive%20system.

tine about 5 ft long.[7] The term "bowel" refers to both the small and large intestines. The large intestine consists of the colon and the rectum, the part that attaches the colon to the anus.

"Peristalsis" is the medical term for the automatic muscular action that sends food through the digestive system.

The digestive system does not produce urine, the urinary system does, the function of which is to filter the blood, with urine being the main byproduct of that filtration.

Food intake, and even its aroma, activates the chemical part of the digestive system. It activates the secretion of saliva in the mouth and the secretion of gastric juices in the stomach where the food is further digested. If the mouth does not water during a meal, then the body is not really ready for the food even though the mind may be, and digestion of that food will be hindered. Some nutritionists claim that well-salivated food is practically half-digested before it gets to the stomach.

Mechanical digestion occurs as the teeth grind and masticate the food. Chewing breaks down food into smaller particles which are easier to digest.

An old saying is: "Chew your food, your stomach has no teeth." Many nutritionists recommend chewing food until it is liquified in the mouth.

The chemical part of digestion breaks down carbohydrates, fats and proteins (macronutrients) into smaller components that can be

---

[7] https://www.healthline.com/health/digestive-health/how-long-are-your-intestines#small-intestines-length.

utilized by the cells of the body for energy, maintenance, growth and repair. It turns food into microscopic particles that can be absorbed into the bloodstream and sent throughout the body to where they are needed to support physiological function.

The job of digestion is not finished until the food passes through the small and large intestines and the waste is eliminated. Different types of foods cause the secretion of different types of gastric juices in the stomach, some being more acidic, some less acidic. This can become a problem when foods are combined. Now, this is a crucial point: if we eat foods that cause more alkaline (less acidic) gastric juices for their digestion together with foods that require acidic gastric juices for their digestion, the gastric juices combine and tend to null each other out, resulting in food in the stomach that is difficult to digest. It leads to a variety of complications, such as increased digestions times, stomachaches, headaches and fermentation, and, as the food passes through the intestines, putrefaction, gas and breeding of parasites.

In addition, drinking water or other fluids during a meal is not wise, for it dilutes the gastric juices, making them less effective and slowing down the time required for digestion.

Different foods require different digestion times.

Simple and complex carbohydrates digest completely in the small intestine.[8] But not so for high protein, high fat foods such as meat and dairy products and eggs. While the digestion of carbs begins in the mouth when foods are chewed, fat digestion does not begin until it reaches the small intestine, into which bile from the liver is secreted, as explained below.

---

[8] https://www.gutsense.org/gutsense/constipation.html.

Fat molecules are more complex than protein molecules and carb molecules, and the more complex food molecules are, the more effort it takes to digest them. Fats, including oils used for cooking, take longer to digest than other foods. Saturated fat is solid at room temperature, oils are liquid, but both do not mix with water.

The liquid oils we use for cooking have been hydrogenated, turning them into trans fat, a man-made food substance which is not found in nature. Trans fats are not assimilated by the body, because they block normal biochemistry.[9]

Some fats are beneficial to health since they help cells multiply and grow, and keep the body warm. They're the fats found in natural foods, such as avocados, nuts, coconut oil and fish. But saturated fats and trans fats harm the body. Research has shown that both fats (saturated and trans) are deadly to the human organism, causing atherosclerosis, heart disease, and all the inflammatory diseases, such as arthritis, eczema, Irritable Bowel Syndrome (IBS), etc.[10]

Food Transit Time

Many books about constipation tells us that certain foods cause constipation, but they do not adequately explain why. The explanation is that different types of foods require, as stated before, different digestion times.

For example, an apple is almost completely digested in the stomach in about an hour; oranges, grapefruit, bananas and grapes eaten as mono-meals take even less time, about half an

---

[9] Elizabeth Lipski, Ph.D., CCN, <u>Digestive Wellness</u>.
[10] Ibid.

hour.[11] Fats and oils take much longer because fat digestion is a complex process involving not only the mouth and stomach, but also the pancreas, liver, and small intestines. Fats/oils are separated from other food substances in the stomach, but not digested until they reach the small intestines as the bile secreted into them from the liver together with the enzymes from the pancreas emulsifies them.

"The foods that take the longest to digest are fats; they can last in the stomach [alone] up to 8 to 10 hours at times. Oils are considered fats. Carbohydrates are usually the first to be digested followed by proteins." - Dr. Michael Fidanzato, Gastroenterologist.[12]

It is typically said that meat and fish digest in 2-3 days due to their complex fat and protein molecules.[13] However, according to accredited sources, it typically takes longer than that for meat and fish to be digested.[14] [15]

A 2021 article entitled, *"How Long Does It Take to Digest a Pizza?"*, states that 6 to 8 hours are required for just the stomach to digest pizza.[16] It is what gives us that full, bloated feeling after eating pizza.

---

[11] https://www.donat.com/how-long-does-it-take-to-digest-food/#:~:text=On%20digesting%20fruit&text=Its%20cousins%2C%20melons.
[12] https://www.findatopdoc.com/Questions/what-foods-take-the-longest-to-digest.
[13] https://www.reference.com/science/long-digest-fish-3082c2c28cffb5df.
[14] Additionally, the article includes an interesting breakdown of what happens to the brain after ingesting a Big Mac at 10, 20, 30, 40 and 60 minute intervals.
[15] https://www.sciencealert.com/here-s-what-eating-a-big-mac-does-to-your-body-in-an-hour.
[16] https://health.clevelandclinic.org/how-long-does-it-take-to-digest-food/#:~:text.

The Only Cure for Constipation

Simple carbohydrates, such white bread, rice and pasta, take 30-60 minutes to pass from the stomach. But if you put add peanut butter on toast, or avocado on eggs, it can take more than four hours just to leave the stomach.[17]

The takeaway is that constipation is mainly caused by foods that require long digestion times. Infrequent bowel movements, which is typically how constipation is defined,[18] [19] [20] are caused by foods that have long digestion times. This is important to understand if you want to cure yourself of constipation.

Our lives depend on the proper functioning of the digestive system. But when we do something that adversely affects the functioning of the body, such as eating foods that are hard to digest in all the organs of the GI tract, and combining foods improperly as is typically done in the Western diet, we suffer the consequences, and one of them is constipation. That big meal you had four or five days ago has not been expelled, and meanwhile you have ingested food that gets congested in the intestines because it has no place to go until that former big meal is expelled, so what happens? The waste gets compacted and becomes a blockage that worsens the situation in the ways described in this book, and it keeps building on itself as time goes by.

We all brush our teeth to feel clean after a meal. Take it a step further and cleanse your GI tract by eating foods for health.

---

[17] Ibid.
[18] https://www.consumerreports.org/constipation/best-drugs-for-constipation-a7214448972/.
[19] https://www.mayoclinic.org/diseases-conditions/constipation/symptoms-causes/syc-20354253#:~:text=Constipation%.
[20] https://my.clevelandclinic.org/health/diseases/4059-constipation.

Chapter 2 The American/Western Diet

The Standard American, or Western, diet consists of high intakes of cooked foods, including meats, dairy products, eggs, refined grain products, jarred, canned and bottled fruits and vegetables, fractionated oils, refined sugar and refined salt. The diet is known to cause many of the diseases and health issues that are prevalent in the world today.[21]

While whole (uncooked, unprocessed) fruits and vegetables are the optimum sources of nutrients for the human body,[22] many people do not eat these foods.

Many food advertisements contribute to the indoctrinated belief that meat and dairy products, sugary foods and drinks, and refined and processed foods, are good for us, and many people keep eating them even after they have a disease. However, according to USDA's Dietary Guidelines for Americans, the average American diet consists of excess salt, saturated fat, refined grains, and added sugars,[23] and the average American intake of fresh vegetables and fruits has dropped dramatically while our use of very cheap animal meats has risen.[24]

Our epidemic of obesity and diabetes, and the ever-increasing incidence of colon cancer, diverticulosis and other diseases that have been tied to modern diets is no coincidence, as many nutri-

---

[21] https://www.webmd.com/digestive-disorders/what-your-gut-bacteria-say-your-health.
[22] https://www.healthline.com/nutrition/improve-gut-bacteria.
[23] https://www.dietaryguidelines.gov/sites/default/files/2020-12/Dietary_Guidelines_for_Americans_2020-2025.pdf.
[24] https://www.gicare.com › GI Health Resources.

tionists and nutrition-minded medical doctors and researchers contend. It is also no coincidence that urgent care centers in this country have become as numerous and widespread as fast-food restaurants.

We need look no further for proof of the destructiveness of most of most diets than the rising incidence of heart disease, cancer, kidney disease, diabetes and a host of other life-shortening sicknesses, some of which were unknown only a few decades ago. The same is true for the joint-related diseases, such as arthritis, bursitis, ankylosing spondylitis, avascular necrosis and gout. All are on the rise in this country and in the world.

The firm conviction of many nutritionists is that nothing that man can do to foods, such as high temperature heat treatment, the addition of preservatives, artificial colors and flavors, the host of chemicals discussed above, antibiotics (in animal products), and other refined and/or man-made ingredients, can improve the food value of the foods over their living food counterparts.

My interest in foods and nutrition has spanned over 30 years. I have witnessed the decline of health in this country and the erosion of the quality of life that people suffer who have been stricken with dangerous diseases, as well as various other health issues, because of the many health hazards associated with commonly eaten foods.

I was raised on, and for years ate the Standard American Diet, until I realized the harm it was doing to me and those around me, not only in terms of constant headaches, heartburn and all the other symptoms of ill health, but more severe harm. It was then that I began to study and learn all I could about foods and nutrition, and about how to put into practice what I had learned. Hopefully, this book will pass some of that knowledge onto others.

Chapter 3 Common GI Problems

Common gastrointestinal (GI) problems plaque most people in the world.[25] They include not only constipation, but many other diseases that result from constipation or are due to supplementary causes. But the common factor in them all is diet, the foods that are eaten.

Because most people are not familiar with medical terms used for constipation and other GI problems, health issues are often shrouded in mystery, which, of course, doesn't help those who want to avoid or rid themselves of them. It behooves us, therefore, to learn something about this terminology. The reader is referred to the footnoted references for additional information.

Chronic Constipation

As discussed in the chapter on The Digestive System, constipation is typically defined medically as having fewer than three bowel movements a week. [26] [27] [28] In the literature, both medical and non-medical, chronic (long-term) constipation and constipation (without the chronic prefix) are generally considered the same thing, since both terms commonly mean having fewer than three bowel movements a week, and both are used to describe the condition whereby a person has an urge to defecate but, when sitting on the toilet, nothing comes out. The time factor is of

---

[25] https://www.medicalnewstoday.com/articles/314059.
[26] https://www.consumerreports.org/constipation/best-drugs-for-constipation-a7214448972/.
[27] https://www.mayoclinic.org/diseases-conditions/constipation/symptoms-causes/syc-20354253#:~:text=Constipation%.
[28] https://my.clevelandclinic.org/health/diseases/4059-constipation.

particular importance in making a person susceptible to serious diseases other than constipation.

However, despite the medically accepted definition of a constipated condition, a person is constipated if they are having more than three bowel movements a week and passing hard and difficult-to-defecate stools.

Bowel movements are considered normal if feces are soft -- but not loosely soft or liquid as diarrhea -- normal sized, and pass easily out of the system.[29]

For healthy, unconstipated people, who eat no oils, meat, dairy or bread products, all of which are known to cause constipation, it is normal to have at least three bowel movements *per day*,[30] or one about every 8 hours. In reality, however, since we tend to eat large meals, and it typically takes 2-3 or more expulsions for the solid wastes of a single meal to pass, a healthy person should have a bowel movement about every 4 hours. Since there are 24 hours in a day, it means having 24/4, or 4 bowel movements per day. If you count back to when each meal was taken, it typically means a total food transit time from mouth to toilet of 54-62 hours.

In any case, it tells us that if we knew how to speed up our bowel movements, not artificially or temporarily by using drugs or other medical means, but hopefully naturally, then we would know something about how to cure constipation, for what goes in must come out, except for the liquids and nutrients that are internally absorbed.

According to the International Foundation for Gastrointestinal

---

[29] https://www.mass.gov/files/documents/2016/07/ol/hpci-risk-constipation.pdf.
[30] Elizabeth Lipski, Ph.D., CCN, Digestive Wellness.

The Only Cure for Constipation

Disorders, nearly everyone has at least three bowel movements per week,[31] which is way too long for good health and much too long for optimum health, and for some people it can be much longer, sometimes more than a week before they have a single bowel movement, which only worsens a constipated condition and leads to other GI problems.

Fecal impaction, aka bowel impaction, is a form of chronic constipation. It occurs when a large, rock-hard mass of stool gets stuck in the colon or rectum that cannot be pushed out. The problem can be so severe that it can cause death.[32] [33]

A 2017 Statnews article reveals that as feces linger in the colon, water is continuously absorbed from them. While this makes feces smaller, it also makes them harder.

"During the first week of my internship, I was working in the intensive care unit when a frail elderly woman was admitted after she had a heart attack. As I was trying to figure out what had caused it, I pressed on her belly and felt something hard. We immediately got an X-ray, which revealed that she had a fecalith – a stone-like mass of stool lodged in her colon. Fecaliths, particularly those as large as hers, are removed surgically, but my patient died before that could happen." - H. J. Warraich, Cardiologist.[34]

Chronic constipation is the most common GI problem in the US. It is estimated that very few people in the world live without it.[35]

---

[31] https://iffgd.org/resources/publication-library/what-is-constipation-anyway/.
[32] https://www.webmd.com/digestive-disorders/what-is-fecal-impaction#:~:text=If%20you%27ve%20been%20constipated,problem%20may%20be%20life-threatening.
[33] https://www.statnews.com/2017/08/17/constipation-bowels-colon/.
[34] https://www.statnews.com/2017/08/17/constipation-bowels-colon/.
[35] https://www.ncbi.nlm.nih.gov/pmc/articles/PMC6503315/.

However, most statistics on constipation belie this truth, or else give it a wide range of occurrence. For example, a 2018 NIH National Library of Medicine article concluded that the prevalence of constipation among the populace is 16%, although it ranges up to 79%.[36] More stats are given below.

We learned in the chapter on The Digestive System that the main causes of constipation are foods that require long digestion times, which, as noted throughout this book, are typically the foods that are most commonly eaten in the American or Western style diet. Less frequent causes of constipation are neurological problems, hormone problems, pregnancy, etc.[37] [38]

Chronic Constipation Symptoms

Symptoms commonly attributed to chronic constipation include the following. [39] [40] [41]

Fatigue
Bloated feeling in the abdomen
Difficulty passing stool and urge to strain during the process
Distended or swollen anus (one that protrudes or juts out more than normal)
Headaches

---

[36] https://www.ncbi.nlm.nih.gov/pmc/articles/PMC5976340/#:
[37] https://www.mayoclinic.org/diseases-conditions/constipation/symptoms-causes/syc20354253#:~:text=Being%20dehydrated,medications%.
[38] https://www.bangkokhospital.com/en/content/constipation.
[39] https://www.mayoclinic.org/diseases-conditions/constipation/symptoms-causes/.
[40] https://www.consumerreports.org/constipation/best-drugs-for-constipation-a7214448972/.
[41] https://bellalindemann.com/blog/side-effects-of-constipation#:~:text=Effects%20of%20constipation%20on%20FATIGUE&text=A%20lack%20of%20healthy%20flora,energy%20levels%20and%20cause%20fatigue.

Sores in the mouth
Blood in stools

Of course, another sign or symptom of chronic constipation is the time it takes for food to travel from the mouth through the anus, although it is not cited as a symptom in the medical literature. The reason it is not cited is probably because most people, including medical doctors, do not know how to measure it. There is, however, a very simple way to measure GI tract transit time, which helps in measuring bowel transit time. It is given in Chapter 12.

A 2013 American Gastroenterological Association Web article stated that, *based on visits to clinicians*, about 16% of adults have the symptoms of constipation, and about 33% 60 years and older have the symptoms.[42]

A 2020 American Journal of Gastroenterology (AJG) article concluded that 37% of Americans aged 18 years or older who experienced constipation discussed their symptoms with a doctor or other clinician, including a primary care provider or gastroenterologist.[43] And it is typically cited in the medical literature that at least 2.5 million people see a doctor each year because of constipation. But how many people who suffer from the condition ever see a doctor, or are part of a survey conducted on constipation? Very few I presume. The fact that mainstream medicine is not able to cure any of the common GI problems may make most people choose to remedy them on their own or live with them without seeing a doctor. In comparison, only a third of the roughly

---

[42] https://www.niddk.nih.gov/health-information/digestive-diseases/constipation/definition-facts#:.
[43] https://journals.lww.com/ajg/fulltext/2020/06000/chronic_constipation.

10 million people with hemorrhoids in the US seek medical treatment for them.[44]

The above sources make chronic constipation, statistically, a rarely occurring malady despite its apparent universal prevalence.

It should be remembered that constipation increases the risk of getting even more serious diseases. For example, clogged up wastes in the colon and rectum are known to cause, or contribute to, colon cancer, heart disease, kidney disease and brain disease.[45] [46] [47] [48] [49]

Because of the hard, impacted wastes, straining is required for expulsion, which can cause hemorrhoids (hemorrhoidal disease) anal fissures (tears in the lining of the anus), and other complications.[50] [51] [52]

Cancers of the GI Tract

Cancers of the GI tract are common throughout the world, and particularly in the US. When detected at an early stage, which is typically not the case, medical treatments are more effective.

---

[44] https://www.mayoclinic.org/medical-professionals/digestive-diseases/news/hemorrhoidal-disease-diagnosis-and-management/mac-20430067.
[45] https://www.ncbi.nlm.nih.gov/pmc/articles/PMC6503315/.
[46] https://www.bangkokhospital.com/en/content/constipation.
[47] https://www.mass.gov/files/documents/2016/07/ol/hpci-risk-constipation.pdf.
[48] https://www.ncbi.nlm.nih.gov/pmc/articles/PMC6503315/.
[49] https://www.hopkinsmedicine.org/health/wellness-and-prevention/gastrointestinal-issues-whats-your-brain-have-to-do-with-it.
[50] https://www.bangkokhospital.com/en/content/constipation.
[51] https://www.mayoclinic.org/medical-professionals/digestive-diseases/news/hemorrhoidal-disease.
[52] https://www.mayoclinic.org/diseases-conditions/anal-fissure/symptoms-causes/syc-20351424.

Cancer is known as a *silent killer* because it does its deadly work without giving any obvious signs or symptoms until it reaches a malignant stage, for until tumors have formed it is rarely properly diagnosed. In other words, it takes a tumor in one of the organs before cancer can be diagnosed correctly by doctors and treated either through surgery and drugs, or chemotherapy.[53] It is why the American Cancer Society recommends routine GI tract cancer screenings start as early as age 45.[54]

The most common types of gastrointestinal cancers are: [55] [56]

1) Esophagus (esophageal) cancer
2) Stomach (gastric) cancer
3) Pancreas (pancreatic) cancer
4) Liver cancer, and
5) Colon or rectum (colorectal) cancer

While medical science searches for the answers, it is well known, as stated previously, that there is a direct link between these cancers and the foods that are commonly consumed.[57]

Esophageal Cancer

The cells in the lining of the esophagus secrete mucus-like fluids

---

[53] https://www.dignityhealth.org/conditions-and treatments/oncology/gastrointestinal-cancer.
[54] https://www.cancer.org/cancer/colon-rectal-cancer/detection-diagnosis-staging/acs-recommendations.html.
[55] https://www.yalemedicine.org/conditions/gastrointestinal-cancers.
[56] https://www.cancer.gov/publications/dictionaries/cancer-terms/def/biliary-system.
[57] See the books cited in the Bibliography for additional information.

to help move swallowed food into the stomach. Cancer can develop in these cells, forming tumors. Symptoms include trouble swallowing, hiccups, pain in throat, and blood in the vomit.[58] Esophageal cancer is rare in the US, amounting to about 1% of cancers, but it is more prevalent in the rest of the world.

Stomach Cancer

Stomach cancer is one of the most common of all cancers. It develops when tumors form in the lining of the stomach.[59] It is known that diets high in meat and processed foods, and low in vegetables, are the major risk factors for stomach cancer.

Steve McQueen of Hollywood fame died of heart failure while recovering from surgery to remove cancerous tumors of the stomach and neck.[60] As recorded in Grady Ragsdale Jr.'s book, *Steve McQueen, the Final Chapter*, his main diet, even when in hospital, was cheeseburgers, fries and a Coke (typically smuggled in). Like other cancers, symptoms arise when the disease has spread to malignancy. They may include abdominal pain, dark stools or blood in the stools.[61]

As explained in this book, how the body wards off health issues, such as common GI problems, is dependent in large part on what a person eats and what they refrain from eating.

---

[58] https://www.cancer.gov/pediatric-adult-rare-tumor/rare-tumors/rare-digestive-system-tumors/esophageal.
[59] https://www.hopkinsmedicine.org/health/conditions-and-diseases/stomach-gastric-cancer.
[60] https://www.elpasotimes.com/story/news/2020/11/04/steve-mcqueen-last-chance-surgery-dies-juarez-due-cancer/3751114001/.
[61] https://www.hopkinsmedicine.org/health/conditions-and-diseases/stomach-gastric-cancer.

Pancreatic Cancer

Pancreatic cancer is an aggressive and highly malignant cancer that is the third leading cause of death in the US, ranking after cancers of the lung and colon.[62] Typical of other cancers, it is usually diagnosed only in advanced stages.

"Diagnosis of early stage pancreatic cancer is even more of a challenge as these tumors may be missed on imaging."[63]

Greater than 90% of pancreatic cancer are adenocarcinoma, or malignant tumor cancer.[64]

Liver cancer

Liver cancer is the most rapidly rising cancer in the US.[65] It is not to be confused with cirrhosis of the liver, although most people with cirrhosis of the liver also have liver cancer.[66] It is typically caused by hepatitis B virus (HBV) or hepatitis C virus (HCV).[67]

Colon Cancer

Colon cancer, also called colorectal cancer (medically termed "CRC"), is the second leading cause of death in the US,[68] and the

---

[62] https://www.cdc.gov/cancer/dcpc/research/update-on-cancer-deaths/index.htm.
[63] https://www.ncbi.nlm.nih.gov/pmc/articles/PMC5051149/.
[64] https://www.ncbi.nlm.nih.gov/books/NBK562137/.
[65] https://www.ncbi.nlm.nih.gov/pmc/articles/PMC7001577/.
[66] https://my.clevelandclinic.org/health/diseases/15572-cirrhosis-of-the-liver#:~:text=No%2C%20cirrhosis%20of%20the%20liver,diseases%20often%20lead%20to%20cirrhosis.
[67] https://www.cancer.org/cancer/types/liver-cancer/causes-risks.
[68] https://www.cdc.gov/cancer/dcpc/research/update-on-cancer-deaths/index.htm.

third most common cancer in men and women in the world (after breast and lung cancers).[69]

It occurs when colon polyps grow in the colon or rectum and become cancerous. Since colon cancer is a silent killer and the symptoms of which do not manifest themselves for years, it is typically detected in diagnostic screening, for example by colonoscopy, which involves inserting a long, flexible tube with a tiny camera at the end through the rectum. When detected, doctors typically advise the surgical removal of the cancerous parts of the body. Other medical treatments include radiation therapy and chemotherapy.[70]

"The value of medical examinations is not to be underestimated – but in a majority of cases, result rather than the cause is given more consideration by the examining physician." - Dr. Benedict Lust, *Overcoming Constipation Naturally*.[71]

Bear in mind that invasive procedures carry many risks. For example, of the total screenings done for colon cancer each year, some 70,000 (0.5%) people are killed or injured in colonoscopy related complications, which is 22% more than the total number of annual deaths from colon cancer itself.[72] [73]

It means that if you undergo a colonoscopy, which, itself, does not involve many of the hazards of a surgical procedure, your chances

---

[69] https://www.wcrf.org/cancer-trends/worldwide-cancer-data/
[70] https://www.mayoclinic.org/diseases-conditions/colon-cancer/diagnosis-treatment/drc-20353674#.
[71] Part of the book: Arnold Ehret's The Definite Cure of Chronic Constipation.
[72] https://www.acpjournals.org/doi/10.7326/0003-4819-145-12-200612190-00004.
[73] Konstantin Monastyrsky, How to Prevent Nutritional Disorders and Premature Aging with Functional Nutrition.

of dying from colon cancer are higher than if you had not gone in for the examination.

Colon cancer and rectal cancer are closely related because the colon and rectum are attached to each other. The cancer is known to cause a gut barrier dysfunction known as "leaky gut syndrome."

Like all cancers, colon cancer lowers the body's defensive mechanisms, which can make the body susceptible to viruses and other microbes, such as COVID-19 and its many variants.

Medical science is mystified about what actually causes colon cancer. It is evidenced by the vast amount of literature on colon cancer medical research in books and articles. Instead of rooting out the cause or causes, it attributes the disease to its symptoms, such as tumors, which, however, are not the underlying causes.[74] [75]

A close relation of mine died in agony of colon cancer at the early age of 57. A favorite breakfast of hers was a cheese omelet with buttered toast (a typical American-style breakfast), which exemplified much of what else she ate. She saw no harm in these things since they're tasty and are served in restaurants, and since all ingredients are sold in food stores. I'm sure many people know a friend or family member whose life was similarly cut short by some kind of cancer.

The chief role of medical research is analyzing and classifying

---

[74] https://www.dignityhealth.org/conditions-and treatments/oncology/gastrointestinal-cancer.
[75] https://www.dignityhealth.org/conditions-and treatments/oncology/gastrointestinal-cancer.

minutiae of information about health disorders, which contributes greatly to it missing the big picture. Mainstream medicine is rooted in the reductionist paradigm, a way of thinking that everything can be understood through its component parts.

"When you're looking through a microscope, either literally or metaphorically, you can't see the big picture." - T. Colin Campbell and Howard Jacobson, *Whole, Rethinking the Science of Nutrition.*

"The synthesis and ultimate unity of all phenomena have therefore been lost under the plethora of minutiae."[76]

The underlying cause of colon cancer is not a mystery to nutritionists, such as those who are referenced in this book, who claim that it is mainly caused by faulty diet, such as a low fiber diet, together with little or no physical activity. Unlike the approach used by mainstream medicine research to understand disease, nutritionists employ the wholistic approach, which is based on how the various component parts of the body work together, which is in line with how Nature operates. Nature works in wholistic ways, with all parts working together, never with one part working on its own.

An old saying seems to be apropos here, "You can't see the forest for the trees." We cannot see the forest when we are focusing on the trees. To solve the problems of diseases you must to have a wholistic view of what causes them and what needs to be done to cure them.

Again, it is extremely important to realize that a constipated condition can increase the risks of getting GI tract cancers.[77][78]

---

[76] Callum Coats, Living Energies.

The Only Cure for Constipation

"Constipation and certain cancers may be independently classified, but they are convergent diseases caused by common underlying risk factors, with a longer latency period for clinically detectable cancer." - Jens Sundbøll, et al, Department of Clinical Epidemiology, Aarhus University Hospital, Denmark.[79]

Constipation is also implicated in the development of heart disease.[80] These things make constipation not just an ordinary health risk as many believe it is, but a risk to life itself. They strongly challenge us to do our utmost to cure constipation.

Symptoms of GI Tract Cancers

Symptoms commonly attributed to GI tract cancers include the following.[81] [82] [83]

Constipation
Abdominal cramping or pain
Rectal bleeding
Difficulty swallowing
Fatigue
Digestive problems
Jaundice
Nausea and vomiting
Swelling in the abdomen

---

[77] https://www.sciencedaily.com/releases/2012/10/121022081228.htm#:~:text=Researchers%20found%20that%3A&text=Both%20colorectal%20cancer%20.
[78] https://www.ncbi.nlm.nih.gov/pmc/articles/PMC6503315/.
[79] Ibid.
[80] https://www.ncbi.nlm.nih.gov/pmc/articles/PMC6399019/.
[81] https://patient.gastro.org/colorectal-cancer-crc/
[82] https://www.yalemedicine.org/conditions/gastrointestinal-cancers.
[83] https://www.cancer.gov/publications/dictionaries/cancer-terms/def/biliary-system.

Weight loss, or loss of appetite

These symptoms are shared with a variety of other health issues and, therefore, cannot be relied on to indicate the actual presence of cancer, making medical diagnosis necessary as previously stated. Fatigue, for example, especially in the mornings, can be due to congested wastes caused by constipation.[84] Hindering the body's ongoing efforts to detoxify itself of toxic substances that enter the bloodstream may also negatively impact energy levels and cause fatigue.

Diverticulitis and Diverticulosis

Both terms refer to a disease of the large intestine (colon) that arises when small pockets or bulges, called diverticula, form on the inner walls of the colon. As their "itis" endings suggest, they are inflammatory diseases. When the bulges become inflamed or infected, the condition is called diverticulitis.[85] Diverticulosis occurs when the diverticula push outward through weak spots in the wall of the colon. [86] [87] [88] The conditions are said to be age related, and that half of all people between the ages of 60 and 80 have diverticular disease.[89]

"When the intestinal lining is damaged even more, substances

---

[84] https://bellalindemann.com/blog/side-effects-of-constipation#:~:text=Effects%20of%20constipation%20on%20FATIGUE&text=A%20lack%20of%20healthy%20flora,energy%20levels%20and%20cause%20fatigue.

[85] https://my.clevelandclinic.org/health/diseases/10352-diverticular-disease.

[86] https://www.mayoclinic.org/diseasesconditions/diverticulitis/symptoms-causes/syc-20371758#.

[87] Elizabeth Lipski, Ph.D., CCN, Digestive Wellness.

[88] https://www.niddk.nih.gov/health-information/digestive-diseases/diverticulosis-diverticulitis/definition-facts#diverticulitis.

89 https://www.mayoclinic.org/diseases-conditions/constipation/symptoms-causes/syc20354253#:~:text=Being%20dehydrated,medications%20to%20lowe.

larger than particle size (disease-causing bacteria, potentially toxic molecules and undigested food particles) are passed directly through the weakened cell membranes. They go directly into the bloodstream...It is the basis for a condition called increased intestinal permeability, or leaky gut syndrome" - Elizabeth Lipski, Ph.D., CCN, *Digestive Wellness*.

Both are bowel dysfunctions that are not prevalent in healthy people and are indicative of poor dietary practices.[90][91] According to the American Society of Colon & Rectal Surgeons, diverticular disease is more common in people who eat little fiber.[92]

Diverticulitis can cause severe constipation accompanied by abdominal pain, fever and nausea. Severe or recurring diverticulitis requires surgery.

Crohn's Disease

Crohn's disease is a type of inflammatory bowel disease that can affect any part of the gastrointestinal tract. It is said to be an autoimmune disease whereby the immune system attacks the digestive tract by mistake.[93] It causes abdominal pain, diarrhea, fatigue, weight loss and anemia.[94][95]

Hemorrhoids

Hemorrhoids are swollen veins in the lower rectum or anus. They

---

[90] Herbert M. Shelton, Superior Nutrition.
[91] Elizabeth Lipski, Ph.D., CCN, Digestive Wellness.
[92] https://www.livestrong.com/article/464063-what-foods-contain-cellulose/.
[93] https://intermountainhealthcare.org/ services/gastroenterology/conditions.
[94] https://www.mayoclinic.org/diseases-conditions/crohns-disease/symptoms-causes/syc-20353304#:~
[95] https://en.wikipedia.org/wiki/Crohn%27s_disease.

are the common result of a constipated condition, and occur when the veins become pushed out due to hard stools.[96] They can cause rectal bleeding (blood on toilet paper), pain during bowel move-ments and intense anal itching. According to website articles, 75% of people experience hemorrhoids at some time in their lives, and is a much better indicator of the prevalence of constipation that what we have seen in general medical statistics.

If the anus itches mainly at night, then you may have pinworms. To check, place a piece of tape around the fingers sticky side out and put it on the anus. When you pull it off, check for worms which look like "moving white threads."[97]

For obvious reasons, seldom do people talk about hemorrhoids, much less visit a doctor to discuss its relief, but prefer, like they do with constipation, to suffer in silence while trying to remedy the condition by using treatments such as witch hazel or Preparation H.

"Many patients with hemorrhoids only seek medical care when they're tired of dealing with them," - Dr. Sarah B. Umar, M.D., Gastroenterologist, Mayo Clinic.[98]

However, like constipation, the underlying problem must be dealt with before the hemorrhoids go away. In almost all cases, hemorrhoids disappear after eliminating the foods that cause them, but most people do not know this fact, or they're convinced they're already eating a healthy diet and do not want to change it, even though meat and cheese contribute to hardening of the arteries,

---

[96] Ever wonder why people use the word "shit" when frustrated or disgusted?
[97] Ibid.
[98] https://www.mayoclinic.org/medical-professionals/digestive-diseases/news/hemorrhoidal-disease-diagnosis-and-management/mac-20430067.

constipation, and hard to eliminate stools. So, they use salves and lotions and take Sitz baths instead.

Hemorrhoids are one of the most painful afflictions people can get. It is said that Napoleon lost the Battle of Waterloo because he could not stay on his horse long enough to survey the situation of the troops and encourage his men to victory – due to his very painful hemorrhoids. Anyone who has had hemorrhoids can testify to the extent of the pain and discomfort they can cause. I would not have even considered getting on a horse, much less riding one, with the hemorrhoids I had. It's a terrible affliction!

It is generally believed that foods high in fiber with plenty of fluids taken during the day to compensate is a cure-all for hemorrhoids and constipation. High fiber foods include wholegrain breads like wheat, rye and barley. But what is not commonly known is that if too much fiber is eaten, especially like the coarse German-bread variety, and not enough fluids are taken, then it is difficult for the fiber to be fully digested and expelled. In addition, the starch in bread begins its deadly work (as will be seen later) as soon as it reaches the intestines, which worsens a constipated condition.

Even medical treatments such as surgery cannot ensure that hemorrhoids do not return because they do not treat the cause.

About 8 or 9 years ago, I had both internal and external (pro-lapsed) hemorrhoids at the same time. It was not due to the foods that are commonly eaten in America. It was because of the high fiber foods I was eating at the time, including an abundance of beans and wholegrain rye bread I got from a German bakery. I tried everything to cure and lessen the pains, but nothing worked.

Then I discovered the cure, a simple natural condiment known for its curative powers.[99] There have been no hemorrhoids since.

GI Bleeding

Bleeding can occur anywhere in the GI tract, from the mouth to the anus, and it includes rectal bleeding. Signs can be obvious, but they are sometimes hidden.

Symptoms of GI Bleeding

Vomiting blood
Black, tarry stools
Lightheadedness
Difficulty breathing
Fainting
Abdominal pain
Drop in blood pressure
Urinating infrequently
Rapid pulse
Unconsciousness

The bleeding can be the result of cancer of the esophagus, stomach or colon, tears in the esophagus, diverticulosis or diverticulitis, hemorrhoids, ulcerative colitis, peptic ulcers, etc. It's main cause, however, is not any of these conditions, but, again, faulty diet.[100] [101] [102] [103] [104] [105]

---

[99] For the only cure that works on hemorrhoids, see the book, How to Heal Hemorrhoids: A Permanent Cure, by Stan Shepherd.
[100] https://medlineplus.gov/gastrointestinalbleeding.html#.
[101] https://www.niddk.nih.gov/health-information/digestive-diseases/gastrointestinal-bleeding.
[102] Arnold Ehret, The Mucusless Diet Healing System.
[103] Dr. Ann Wigmore, Be Your Own Doctor.

The Only Cure for Constipation

Some websites urge a doctor visit for the condition if it lasts for longer than 1-2 days. However, it typically takes more time than that to get rid of culprit foods that are causing the hard stools, and replace them with foods that remedy the situation. It's best to first adjust the diet before visiting a doctor for in most cases the condition can be remedied naturally without incurring doctor visits.

A typical reaction to blood in stools evidenced by red splotches on toilet paper or red in the toilet bowl is that it must be life-threatening. Indeed, it can be life-threatening if it lasts for weeks on end, but based on my research most of the time it goes away after a few days if the diet is corrected, for its main cause is foods that cause constipation and hard stools.

If a doctor is consulted, the diagnosis may involve invasive procedures, such as a nasogastric lavage, in which the contents of the stomach are vacuumed through a tube inserted into the stomach through the nose. Esophagogastroduodenoscopy (EGD) is another procedure, during which an endoscope, or flexible tube with a small video camera on the end, is inserted through the mouth and esophagus into the stomach and duodenum. As mentioned previously, colonoscopy, which may also be employed to find where the bleeding is from, is a medical procedure that involves inserting a long, flexible tube with a tiny camera at the end through the rectum.[106]

Rectal bleeding can be a sign of cancer. If it is cancer, treatment

---

[104] Robert Morse, N.D., The Detox Miracle Sourcebook.
[105] Norman W. Walker, Colon Health.
[106] https://www.webmd.com/digestive-disorders/blood-in-stool, and the links provided therein.

often means surgical removal of the tumors.[107]

Irritable Bowel Syndrome (IBS)

IBS affects the colon. It causes abdominal pain or cramping, gas, bloating, diarrhea and constipation.

Some studies indicate that 10-15% [26 million to 39 million] US adults have IBS, but others estimate 10-20% percent.[108] However, it is reported that only about 7% of US adults are diagnosed with IBS because most people who have it tend to live with the condition, since it usually goes away after a few defecations.[109] [110]

People have been known to see improvement after eliminating grain products from their diets.[111]

Like colon cancer, the causes of IBS are not well understood by medical doctors.[112] However, its main cause is not a mystery to nutritionists and nutrition-mined medical doctors, such as those that are referenced in this book, and the cause once again is improper diet.

Diarrhea

Diarrhea typically means watery bowel movements. While

---

[107] https://my.clevelandclinic.org/health/symptoms/14612-rectal-bleeding#:~:text=Rectal%20bleeding%20is%20a%20symptom,bowl%20or%20in%20your%20stool.
[108] Elizabeth Lipski, Ph.D., CCN, Digestive Wellness.
[109] https://my.clevelandclinic.org/health/diseases/4342-irritable-bowel-syndrome.
[110] Ibid.
[111] Elizabeth Lipski, Ph.D., CCN, Digestive Wellness.
[112] https://www.mayoclinic.org/diseases-conditions/colon-cancer/symptoms-causes/syc-20353669#:~:text=Signs%2.

many people have diarrhea occasionally, prolonged diarrhea is a sign of more serious gastrointestinal problems. Most cases of diarrhea, however, are self-limiting, meaning that after a few days without any treatment the problem goes away.

Diarrhea is one of the signs the body gives as it attempts to rid itself of its morbidity through its self-cleansing, self-healing powers. It should not be looked on as a symptom needing drugs to mask it or make the symptoms go away, but as a beacon of warning that something is wrong with the diet.

Dysbiosis

As stated in the chapter on Bacteria in the Gut, dysbiosis is often defined as an imbalance of gut microbiota due to a gain or loss of microbes that thrive in the digestive system.[113][114] Imbalanced gut microbiota are associated with inflammatory disorders and various cancers.[115]

Antibiotics and NSAIDs (Nonsteroidal Anti-inflammatory Drugs) such as Ibuprofen and Aspirin, alter the balance of the gut microbiota,[116] but, as explained in the previous chapter, the imbalance can also be caused by diets high in sugar and low in nutrition.[117][118][119]

---

[113] https://www.drelenaklimenko.com/constipation-relief-part-3-dysbiosis/.
[114] https://www.sciencedirect.com/topics/medicine-and-dentistry/dysbiosis#:~:text=2%20Dysbiosis.
[115] https://www.ncbi.nlm.nih.gov/pmc/articles/PMC6503315/.
[116] Elizabeth Lipski, Ph.D., CCN, Digestive Wellness.
[117] https://www.thegutmicrobiome.com/factors-that-influence-gut-microbiota/.
[118] https://www.hopkinsmedicine.org/health/conditions-and-diseases/constipation.
[119] https://www.phlabs.com/taking-antibiotics-be-sure-to-protect-your-digestive-system.

"Antibiotics simultaneously kill both harmful and helpful bacteria throughout our digestive system, mouth, vagina and skin, leaving the territory to bacteria, parasites, viruses, and yeast that are resistant to the antibiotic that was used." - Elizabeth Lipski, Ph.D., CCN, *Digestive Wellness*.

The imbalance in gut microbiota depletes the body of key minerals and other nutrients that are needed for gastrointestinal health. It is one of the main causes of a weakened immune system (See Appendix III).

A basic instinct of people is to reach for a quick fix when something ails them. But if the pain, inflammation or other discomfort was initially caused by an imbalance of microbes in the gut brought about by poor diet, and the cause was not dealt with by improving the diet, then more toxins will be produced throughout the system, contributing to the pain and inflammation.

Dehydration

Dehydration is caused by not drinking enough water, or fluids that are mostly water and do not dehydrate. It is one of the things that causes constipation and makes stools difficult to pass.[120] [121]

Diuretics dehydrate the body. They also cause the kidneys to flush potassium and magnesium out of the body, thereby causing or contributing to potassium and magnesium deficiency.[122] [123] If you drink a lot of coffee or tea, or if you're on high blood pressure medication, further complications can result. Diuretics can

---

[120] https://www.webmd.com/digestive-disorders/water-a-fluid-way-to-manage-constipation.
[121] https://my.clevelandclinic.org/health/diseases/4059-constipation.
[122] Marietta Whittlesey, Killer Salt.
[123] Sherry A. Rodgers, M.D., The High Blood Pressure Hoax.

damage the kidneys, unless foods high in potassium and magnesium, which include fresh fruits and vegetables, are eaten.[124] Drinking plenty of non-diuretic fluids, such as water, restores bodily fluids.

As mentioned previously, constipation is often called "idiopathic" in the medical literature, which means having an unknown cause, and the fact that the cause of constipation is generally unknown to doctors and other health care professionals is evidenced by how mainstream medicine views constipation – as an affliction that should be treated with drugs. But what do most drugs do? They dehydrate the body.

The cause of many if not most of our health problems, ranging from indigestion and gas to colon cancer to diabetes to heart disease and kidney disease, has been with us for as long as we have lived – the foods that are typically eaten, and, while most people are somewhat aware of this by now, seldom is anything ever done about it except maybe taking drugs at the doctor's advice.

Again, "It is a fact of life is that our diets have changed dramatically in the last 100 years. Our grandmothers would simply not recognize what we now call the Westernized diet. Simply put, food manufacturers and industry now sell "imitation" types of food in boxes, packages and bags, each with dozens of "nutrients" and chemicals added to them. Our intake of fresh vegetables and fruits has dropped dramatically while our use of very cheap animal meats has risen in a similar manner. Additionally, high fructose corn syrup has quietly invaded our lives and

---

[124] For more information, see the book, <u>How to Cure High Blood Pressure</u>, by S. H. Shepherd.

intestinal tracts in soft drinks, packaged foods and almost anywhere a sweetener is used."[125]

It is no coincidence that we are seeing an epidemic of obesity and diabetes, and colon cancer, colon diverticulosis, and other major diseases in the population.

Perforated Colon

A perforated colon is a hole in the colon. It may be caused by a buildup of wastes in the colon that gets stuck, called a bowel impaction. Another cause can be surgery, or procedures used in diagnosing GI tract problems, such as colonoscopy. The hole causes the wastes to leak into the abdomen, which causes infection that can be life threatening.[126] While considered rare, it can and does occur.

Hydrochloric Acid Deficiency

Gastric, or stomach, juices are mainly composed of potassium chloride, sodium chloride, hydrochloric acid. Hydrochloric acid is considered to be the main stomach acid. A deficiency of hydrochloric acid, known as low stomach acid or hypochlorhydria, can occur as a person ages (although I have not seen it happen to me at 73),[127] and cause ingestion and constipation when high protein foods, such as meat and dairy products, are ingested. Also, a diet high in refined and processed foods can cause nutrient deficiency which contributes to hypochlorhydria while depriving the body of important nutrients. [128] [129]

---

[125] https://www.gicare.com/gi-health-resources/prebiotics/.
[126] https://my.clevelandclinic.org/health/diseases/23478-gastrointestinal-perforation.
[127] Victoria Boutenko, Green for Life.
[128] S. H. Shepherd, How to Cure High Blood Pressure.

Low stomach acid can be caused by drugs, such as antacids, or by chronic stress, age, and vitamin and mineral deficiency, including low levels of zinc and thiamine in the bloodstream.[130]

Chapter Summary

Constipation is one of the main causes of a weakened immune system, which means that it is essentially a major contributor to human sickness and disease.

People throughout the world have GI diseases because of clogged up intestinal wastes. While the diseases are, even today, poorly understood by modern science and may require the use of expensive and invasive procedures in order to be diagnosed, they are principally caused by faulty diet, or more specifically by foods that take a long time to pass through the GI tract and which result in infrequent and hard to pass bowel movements. Additionally, many GI diseases, including constipation, are life-threatening.

By choosing to ignore the information that has been gained in the human health field which proves that diseases and a host of lesser human ailments are caused by commonly eaten foods, many of us are sacrificing our health for eating habits and food cravings. But the remarkable truth is that eating habits can be changed, even when food cravings exist, and that everyone is capable of changing their diet in enlightened self-interest.

---

[129] https://www.drelenaklimenko.com/causes-of-constipation-part-1-low-stomach-acid/.
[130] Ibid.

Chapter 4 Standard Treatments for Constipation

For hundreds of years, medical science has focused on achieving health through drugs. For headaches, take Aspirin or a similar product; for stomachaches, take antacids; for infections, take antibiotics; for constipation, take laxatives; for cancer, take chemotherapy or radiation therapy. But even considering drugs like penicillin which can halt the spread of a disease, drugs do not possess the ability to heal, and there are risks associated with all drugs. Also, drugs have been known to lodge in the system for decades after their use.[131]

Medication continues to be the preferred choice of doctors and other health care professionals for treating health issues such as constipation, which is consonant with most people's preference for buying fast foods and drinks, or anything else that saves time so they can get back to doing what they were doing before. In addition, many if not most people are ignorant of the therapeutics that are called alternative medicine, or natural ways of healing.

The standard medical treatments for common GI problems including constipation are based almost entirely on drugs, with medical intervention, such as hospitalization and surgery, because doctors and other health care professionals are rarely trained in the non-pharmacological management of disease.[132] [133] In addition, drugs are typically prescribed by doctors and health care professionals for constipation because, as evidenced in the vast

---

[131] From the book, Prof. Arnold Ehret's Mucusless Diet Healing System: Annotated, Revised, and Edited by Prof. Spira.
[132] Robert E. Kowalski, The Blood Pressure Cure.
[133] Robert Morse, N.D., The Detox Miracle Sourcebook.

amount of literature available on the subject, its cause or causes are said to be unknown, and they are typically attributed entirely to its symptoms, which are what drugs are designed to treat.

To effectively treat any disease, the underlying cause or causes of the disease must be known, or at least acknowledged. Using drugs to treat the disease only masks the symptoms while allowing the underlying causes to progress.

Mainstream medicine has become very dependent on Big Pharma, or you could say that Big Pharma has mainstream medicine in their pocket. If you are currently taking medication for health issues, you are not alone. Two-thirds or 66.7% of all adults in the US take prescription drugs.[134]

According to a 2021 market analysis report, the market for constipation treatment is expected to reach $1.3 billion in 2027, up from $8.5 million in 2019.[135]

Since drugs are so widely for constipation, it is good to learn about them and their side effects.

Drugs Typically Used for Constipation

Because constipation requires change for remedy, and because many people do not know how to effectively remedy their condition on their own, nor do they have the time even if they did know, drugs are commonly taken to temporarily relieve the problem.

---

[134] https://hpi.georgetown.edu/rxdrugs/#:~:text=A%20vital%20component.
[135] https://www.biospace.com/article/constipation-treatment-market-rising-prevalence-of-chronic-constipation/#.

The Only Cure for Constipation

Websites and articles about constipation routinely recommend seeing a doctor for its treatment, and often mention the very drugs that may be prescribed. Some also state that healthy lifestyle changes, such as a change in diet, should be included, but never are they solely recommended, and practically none of websites and articles stress the seriousness or implications of the disease.

The four general types of drugs used for constipation are:

Laxatives
Antacids
Acetaminophen
Aspirin

Each type has proven to be effective for some people in remedying constipation in the short term, but in practice if one type of drug is not found to work well, then another type will be prescribed until a suitable drug, or combination of drugs, is found.

All drugs for constipation are designed to work as though the condition was caused by a deficiency of the medication, which, of course, is not true. As previously discussed, constipation has definite causes that have nothing to do with a deficiency of drugs in the body. It is typically true as well that medication taken for any health disorder or malady is taken on the implicit assumption that the malady exists because of the lack of such medication.

The assumed need for drugs for constipation (or anything else) is a good indicator that the body is in some sort of imbalance.

Even though drugs are standard protocol medical treatment for constipation, independent research has shown that a constipated condition is caused almost invariably by something that a person does or does not do to themselves in the way of what they eat, or

The Only Cure for Constipation

in the way of what they combine to eat. Constipation, like other diseases, may seem to suggest a need for drugs, but it is only because a person does not comply with, or is ignorant of, what is really needed to correct the condition.

The same can also be said for modern drugs that are prescribed for practically any other human illness. Instead of attacking the root cause, or causes, of the affliction, drugs are designed to treat only the symptoms, being palliative in nature rather than curative in nature. And, unfortunately, that is not the whole story, for in addition to their limited efficacy and their inability to cure diseases, drugs have side effects, some of which are serious, and each comes with restrictions or limitations on use, for all drugs are, in some way, harmful to the body. In addition, if used in combination with other drugs, there can be contraindicated drug interactions, some of which can be serious.

Those who are currently using drugs for constipation may notice their particular brand name in the following discussion, but if the medication or side effect is not listed, then refer to the footnoted references for more details.[136] [137] [138] [139] [140] [141] [142] [143] [144] [145] [146] [147]

---

[136] https://www.mayoclinic.org/diseases-conditions/constipation/in-depth/laxatives/art-20045906.

[137] https://www.consumerreports.org/constipation/best-drugs-for-constipation-a7214448972/.

[138] https://www.verywellhealth.com/best-antacids-4171024.

[139] https://spy.com/articles/health-wellness/diet-nutrition/best-antacids-12028.

[140] https://www.amazon.com/Best-Sellers-Acetaminophen/zgbs/hpc/3764011.

[141] https://www.medicalnewstoday.com/articles/is-tylenol-an-nsaid.

[142] https://medlineplus.gov/druginfo/meds/a614018.html.

[143] https://www.mayoclinic.org/drugs-supplements/laxative-oral-route/side-effects/drg-20070683.

[144] https://medlineplus.gov/druginfo/meds/a681004.html#side-effects.

[145] https://www.mercycare.org/healthy-living/health-education/tylenol--advil--when-to-use-which/.

In general, the types of medication typically used to treat constipation act either as purgatives or gastrointestinal stimulants. The purgatives help the bowels retain water which helps move along the wastes. The stimulants increase the motility (contract-ion) of GI muscles to help GI tract contents move along.[148][149] However, no drug is safe for long-term use.

Many websites, such as those cited herein, claim that it is okay to continue eating the way you've always eaten with a bowel movement only once every three days or once a week. In other words, leave it up to the drugs to help you. However, the claim is misleading, for, as explained previously, when constipation-free you will have at least as many bowel movements per day as meals taken per day. It should be the goal of everyone to experience such relief for themselves. It is not a myth, and it is not an unchasable dream. It is simply a rule of nature, and those who abide by Mother Nature's laws experience it.

Laxatives

Laxatives are designed to relieve only occasional constipation. They are typically the first drug to be prescribed, and doctors use them in colon and rectum surgical procedures to help clean out the contents.[150][151] However, like all drugs used for the treatment of constipation, they cannot cure the disease.

---

[146] https://www.rxlist.com/tylenol-side-effects-drug-center.htm#overview.
[147] https://www.drugs.com/aspirin.html.
[148] https://www.healthline.com/health/laxatives-side-effects.
[149] Smooth muscle exists throughout the body. In the urinary system it functions to help purge the body of toxins; in the arteries and veins it helps regulate blood pressure and tissue oxygenation. Ref. https://www.ncbi.nlm.nih.gov/books/NB.
[150] https://www.webmd.com/drugs/2/drug-4385/sodium-phosphates-rectal/.

The Only Cure for Constipation

The main types of laxatives are: bulk, stimulant, osmotic (sometimes called hyperosmotic) and stool softeners. Osmotic laxatives draw water from the body into the bowel. Both bulk and stimulant laxatives help bowel movements by increasing the build, or weight, of the stools and by promoting contraction of the colon muscles. Stool softeners loosen the stool, some by lubricant action as opposed to drawing water from the body into the bowel.[152] [153]

Remember, as previously stated:

"As feces linger in the colon, water is continuously absorbed from them. While this makes feces smaller, it also makes them harder."- Haider J. Warraich, Cardiologist.[154]

Also remember that dehydration (not drinking enough water) is one of the causes of chronic constipation.[155] [156]

Bulk laxatives are generally considered the safest to use, but several days have to pass before they work, and lots of fluids must be taken during that time.[157]

Most OTC (over- the-counter) remedies for constipation are not very helpful, as evidenced by nearly half of users being dissatisfied with their results.[158]

---

[151] https://www.einnews.com/pr_news/586661646/laxative-market-to-witness-huge-growth-by-2029.
[152] https://www.nhs.uk/conditions/laxatives/.
[153] https://www.drugoffice.gov.hk/sps/do/en/customer/news.
[154] https://www.statnews.com/2017/08/17/constipation-bowels-colon/.
[155] https://www.webmd.com/digestive-disorders/water-a-fluid-way-to-manage-constipation.
[156] https://my.clevelandclinic.org/health/diseases/4059-constipation.
[157] Ibid.

The Only Cure for Constipation

Blue Cross Blue Shield estimated in 2022 that Americans spend $725 million per year on laxatives alone. According to a 2022 market analysis report, the laxative market is expected to reach sales of $1.15 Billion by 2029,[159] similar to what was cited previously for all drugs used for constipation, and indicating that laxatives take up the lion's share.

Laxatives are not designed for weight loss. If taken for that purpose, they will not prevent the body from absorbing calories.[160]

Examples of bulk laxatives are psyllium (Metamucil), polycarbophil (FiberCon), methylcellulose (Citrucel) and Fybogel. Examples of stimulant laxatives are Ex-Lax, Senokot, Dr. Schulze's Bowel Flush, Unisex-ZupOO, Feen-a-Mint, castor oil, senna, and phenolphthalein. Examples of osmotic laxatives are CosmoCol and Duphalac (Lactulose). Examples of stool softeners are: Colace, DOK, Dulcolax, Doc-Q-Lac, Miralax, Phillips Laxative Caplets, Fleet laxatives, CVC Stool Softener, mineral oil, olive oil and Milk of Magnesia.

When a particular laxative is not effective, other, typically newer kinds of laxatives are often prescribed. Examples are linaclotide and lubiprostone.[161]

Laxatives are available at local pharmacies and supermarkets. The most popular section at the local pharmacy is the laxative section.

---

[158] https://www.health.harvard.edu/blog/probiotics-may-ease-constipation-201.
[159] https://www.einnews.com/pr_news/586661646/laxative-market-to-witness-huge-growth-by-2029.
[160] https://barnard.edu/self-help-resources/facts-about-laxatives.
[161] https://www.ncbi.nlm.nih.gov/pmc/articles/PMC5976340/#:

The Only Cure for Constipation

Side Effects of Laxatives

Bulk Laxatives

Intestinal blockage
Bloating and flatulence
Abdominal distension
Hypersensitivity
Difficulty in breathing
Difficulty in swallowing
Skin rash

Stimulant Laxatives

Abdominal cramps
Nausea and vomiting
Diarrhea
Local irritation if suppository preparations are used
Fatigue
Confusion
Irregular heartbeat
Muscle cramps

Osmotic Laxatives

Abdominal pain
Bloating and flatulence
Nausea and vomiting
Confusion
Dizziness or light-headedness
Irregular heartbeat
Muscle cramps
Fatigue

Stool Softeners

Dehydration
Stomach pain
Abdominal cramps
Throat irritation (liquid forms only)
Nausea
Increased thirst
Dizziness
Urinating less frequently
Vomiting
Drowsiness
Swelling of the ankles, feet, and legs
Gout

It is important to drink plenty of fluids when taking bulk or osmotic laxatives because dehydration can cause constipation. It suggests that these particular types of laxatives work less effectively than the others.[162]

"Dehydration resulting from laxative abuse can lead to tremors, fainting, weakness, and blurred vision. Severe dehydration can cause organ damage leading to death. Overusing laxatives wears away the protective mucus that lines the colon, leaving the colon susceptible to infections."[163]

Besides the above side effects, overuse of laxatives can cause electrolyte imbalance that interferes with the proper functioning of the nerves and muscles, including those of the heart and blood

---

[162] https://www.nhs.uk/conditions/laxatives/.
[163] Ibid.

vessels, which, according to the literature, can cause urinary tract infections, kidney failure and heart attacks.[164] [165]

An FDA report entitled, "OTC Laxatives Can Harm Kidneys and Heart," confirms cited claims that taking more than a recommended daily dose of laxatives, such as OTC laxatives that contain sodium phosphate, harms the kidneys and heart, increasing the risk of early death.[166] Laxatives that contain sodium phosphate include: stool softeners Colace, DOK, Dulcolax, Doc-Q-Lac, Senokot-S, Miralax, Phillips Laxative Caplets, Fleet laxatives, CVC Stool Softener, and Milk of Magnesia.

Long-term use of laxatives cause the body to rely on them for bowel movements, a condition called *laxative dependence*, which leads to severe constipation and even less frequency of bowel movements.[167] [168] But worse or equally as bad is the fact that long-term use of laxatives can cause infections.[169]

"It is an open secret that all laxatives finally fail, because the constantly overloaded intestines are being over-stimulated by the laxatives and thereby slowly paralyzed. To continually increase the laxatives year after year, instead of changing the diet, means suicide – slow, but sure." - Elizabeth Lipski, Ph.D., CCN, *Digestive Wellness*.

The colon is lined with protective layers of mucus, allowing

---

[164] https://barnard.edu/self-help-resources/facts-about-laxatives#.
[165] https://www.aboutlawsuits.com/fleet-laxatives-may-cause-kidney-heart-injury-fda-58535/.
[166] https://www.empr.com/uncategorized/fda-otc-laxatives-can-harm-kidneys-and aheart/#:~:text=The%.
[167] https://www.webmd.com/drugs/2/drug-4385/sodium-phosphates-rectal/.
[168] https://www.rosewoodranch.com/laxative-abuse-treatment/.
[169] https://www.ncbi.nlm.nih.gov/pmc/articles/PMC3758667/.

bacteria in the colon to do their work in braking down food wastes for cellular maintenance and growth. But long-term laxative use strips away the bacteria and the protective layers of mucus, leaving the body more vulnerable to infection. In addition, studies suggest that long-term laxative use increases the risk of colon cancer.[170]

Reports on the Web relate the effects that people have had when they drinking olive oil. For example, that it takes at least a week for the bowels to return to normal.

Antacids

Antacids help neutralize gastric (stomach) acids to relieve indigestion and heartburn (acid reflux). They come in tablet or liquid form and can be purchased OTC at local supermarkets or pharmacies. Typical ingredients are sodium bicarbonate, calcium carbonate, aluminum hydroxide and magnesium carbonate.

Examples of Antacids are: Prilosec (omeprazole), Rolaids (calcium carbonate), Alka-Seltzer (sodium bicarbonate), Pepto-Bismol (bismuth subsalicylate), Tums (calcium carbonate), Citrical (calcium citrate), Gaviscon (alginic acid), Mylanta, Maalox, and Gelusil (aluminum hydroxide and magnesium carbonate).

It should be remembered that heartburn, stomachache and indigestion are not caused by an antacid deficiency, but primarily by the foods that we eat.

---

[170] https://www.rosewoodranch.com/laxative-abuse-treatment/.

Side Effects of Antacids

Diarrhea
Constipation
flatulence (gas or belching)
stomach cramps
feeling sick, or vomiting
Swelling in the feet, ankles, and hands

When used occasionally, the side effects are minimal and disappear after a day or so, but they are severe and long-term if habitually used.

Antacids are not advised if you have kidney or liver problems, or are on a low-sodium diet, or when taking thyroid medication or blood thinners, since antacids may interfere with these drugs.[171]

Acetaminophen

Acetaminophen is a pain reliever and fever reducer. Some sources claim that Advil and Motrin are acetaminophens, but Advil and Motrin are NSAIDs, or put another way, acetaminophen is not a NSAID,[172] [173] because it does not treat inflammation.

Examples of acetaminophen are: Tylenol Extra Strength (Liquid Gel), CVS Health Extra Strength Acetaminophen Gelcaps, Nyquil, Kroger Pain Relief Extra Strength, Equate Pain Reliever, and Midol Complete.

---

[171] https://www.everydayhealth.com/antacids/guide/.
[172] https://www.mercycare.org/healthy-living/health-education/tylenol--advil--when-to-use-which/.
[173] For a discussion of the side effects of NSAIDs, see the book, The Cure for Arthritis, by S. H. Shepherd.

Side Effects of Acetaminophens

Nausea
Stomach pain
Loss of appetite
Headache
Dizziness
Hoarseness
Difficulty breathing or swallowing
Constipation
Hypersensitivity reactions, skin reactions
Kidney damage
Anemia
Hives
Low platelet count
Liver failure
Peeling or blistering skin, or skin rash
Itching/swelling of the face, throat, tongue, lips, eyes, hands, feet, ankles, or lower legs
Jaundice (yellowing of the skin or eyes)

Constipation is reported to be a side effect of acetaminophens, such as Nyquil.[174] Acetaminophen drugs, such as Tylenol, should not be used for longer than 10 days.[175]

Aspirin

Ancient civilizations, including the Sumerians, Egyptians, Greeks and Romans, used willow bark, which contains a salt or ester of

---

[174] https://www.drugs.com/mtm/nyquil-severe-cold-flu.html.
[175] https://www.mercycare.org/healthy-living/health-education/tylenol--advil--when-to-use-which/.

salicylic acid, as a pain reliever and fever reducer, but now we typically use Aspirin, which has the key ingredient salicylic acid.

Aspirin is a nonsteroidal anti-inflammatory drug (NSAID).[176] It reduces pain and fever, and is anti-inflammatory. It is not an antibiotic, or an antiseptic, so it cannot kill micro-organisms no matter what people believe. It can, however, prevent blood clots, since it is s blood thinner.

Besides Aspirin, NSAIDs include Ibuprofen (Advil, Motrin), Excedrin, Aleve, and also prescription kinds, such as diclofenac, celecoxib (Celebrex), phenylbutazone, and the Corticosteroids, which are hormones that include cortisone, prednisone, and methyl-prednisolone. Tylenol, also used for pain relief, is not a NSAID; rather it is an acetaminophen.

Other examples of Aspirin are: Bufferin, Bayer Aspirin, Kirkland Signature, Vazalore, and St. Joseph Aspirin.

Bufferin is a combination of Aspirin and three antacids: calcium carbonate, magnesium carbonate, and magnesium oxide. Excedrin is a combination of acetaminophen, Aspirin and caffeine, with the caffeine acting as an enhancer.

<u>Side Effects of Aspirin</u>

Nausea
Vomiting
Blood in vomit
Stomach pain
Heartburn

---

[176] https://www.healthline.com/health/pain-relief/is-aspirin-nsaid#nsaid-overview.

Indigestion
Skin rash
Hoarseness
Rapid heartbeat
High blood pressure
Cold, clammy skin
Anemia
Asthma
Hives
Seizure
Ringing in the ears
Loss of hearing
Swelling of the eyes, face, lips, tongue, or throat
Hemophilia
Peptic or stomach ulcers
Liver or kidney disease
Kidney failure
Hemorrhage in the brain or stomach

More Side Effects of Constipation Drugs

Additional side effects besides those listed above for Laxatives, Antacids, Acetaminophen and Aspirin are: ulcers and/or adverse drug reactions.

For example, long-term use of anti-inflammatory drugs like Aspirin, Ibuprofen and naproxen have been known to cause ulcers.[177] [178]

"Constipation – this most common disease – has not decreased or improved in spite of the thousands of remedies for sale on the

---

[177] https://www.nhs.uk/medicines/erythromycin/side-effects-of-erythromycin/.
[178] https://www.webmd.com/digestive-disorders/blood-in-stool.

market, and in spite of so-called medical science; simply, because the "diet of civilization" is unnatural." - Arnold Ehret, *The Definite Cure of Chronic Constipation*.

Additional Treatments for Constipation

Have you ever eaten prunes (dried plums)? Prunes and prune juice have been known for centuries to increase regularity. Prunes contain soluble and insoluble fiber, both of which are discussed in a later chapter. Insoluble fiber helps to remedy constipation because it adds bulk to stools which helps move wastes through the intestines. It is noted that fiber supplements contain only soluble fiber.

Studies have found that prunes cause more frequent bowel movements and better stool consistency than fiber supplements. Other remedies, such as beets or beet supplements (for example, Betafood), increase bile secretion.[179]

However, a better natural treatment may be simply to abstain from or eliminate meat, dairy and grain products from the diet.

According to Consumer Reports, OTC fiber supplements that contain psyllium, such as Metamucil and Konsyl, also reduce constipation.[180]

<u>Drug Recalls</u>

In July 2022, the FDA announced the recall of all flavors of

---

[179] https://www.drelenaklimenko.com/causes-of-constipation-part-2-low-bile-flow/.
[180] https://www.consumerreports.org/medical-conditions/how-to-relieve-constipation/.

The Only Cure for Constipation

Magnesium Citrate Saline Laxatives, including all lots of Cherry Flavored and Grape Flavored Magnesium Citrate Saline Laxative Oral Solution, 10 FL OZ (296 mL) size, due to the presence of gluconacetobacter liquefaciens, which is a bacterium that infects plants and causes spoilage in wine and beer made with plants infected by the bacterium.[181] [182]

In February 2022 and April 2022, various brand named coated and uncoated acetaminophen tablets and caplets 500 mg and less were recalled,[183] [184] cautioning that they could lead to severe liver damage.[185]

The FDA continues to announce recalls on prescription drugs for heartburn, including generic versions of Zantac and another antacid, Nizatidine.[186] For example, a 2020 web article states:

"A cancer-causing substance known as NDMA has been repeatedly found in one of the most popular antacid drugs in the United States [drugs containing Zantac]."[187]

---

[181] https://www.fda.gov/safety/recalls-market-withdrawals-safety-alerts/vi-jon-llc-expands-voluntary-worldwide-recall-all-flavors-and-lots-within-expiry-magnesium-citrate.

[182] https://en.wikipedia.org/wiki/Gluconacetobacter_liquefaciens.

[183] https://www.hmpgloballearningnetwork.com/site/pln/news/acetaminophen-products-recalled#:~:text=Ultra.

[184] https://www.fda.gov/safety/recalls-market-withdrawals-safety-alerts/s-medication-solutions-issues-voluntary-nationwide-recall-acetaminophen-extra-strength-tablets.

[185] https://www.lawyerworks.com/fda-recalls-enteric-coated-aspirin-tablets-due-to-packaging-mistakes/.

[186] https://www.nbcnews.com/health/health-news/fda-announces-more-recalls-antacids-containing-traces-carcinogen-n1113196.

[187] https://www.wired.com/story/the-fda-announces-two-more-antacid-recalls-due-to-cancer-risk/.

Chapter 5 Aging and Constipation

A constipated condition only worsens with age unless changes are made in the diet. It is well known that the older a person gets the more susceptible they become to constipation and an array of other diseases – if one allows their health to decline.

As you get older, the key thing to remember is to drive the body to do what you want to do. You cannot let the body tell you what to do. The body only wants to relax, take it easy and enjoy the foods it has always liked. If it wants to eat a burger, don't let it. You cannot let the body tell you what to do. Health is achieved and sustained by eating foods that have health-appeal over taste-appeal. The lazy body is always ready to give up and quit any health regimen; but not if the mind doesn't want it to. Use the information you have gained from the study of foods and nutrition to guide you into a healthier life. But always remember that success in anything depends on you making it happen. It won't happen just because you want it to happen. You have to make it happen.

Many medical sources tell us that health issues that are more common to seniors, such as stroke, Parkinson's disease, hormone or metabolic dysfunctions like diabetes, pelvic floor disorders, IBS, etc., can cause constipation.[188][189][190] But again, the claims of medical science can differ significantly from the claims of nutritionists, for many nutritionists claim that instead of the medical

---

[188] https://bmcgastroenterol.biomedcentral.com/articles/10.1186/s12876-015-0366-3.
[189] https://www.nia.nih.gov/health/concerned-about-constipation.
[190] https://www.webmd.com/digestive-disorders/features/digestive-health-aging.

conditions themselves causing constipation, the principle cause of constipation, stroke, diabetes, IBS, etc., is improper diet.

A 2023 article on the Web, one that is more in line with what nutritionists have claimed for years, revealed that comparative clinical studies conclude that constipation and other digestive disorders doubles the chances of getting Parkinson's disease, and that the origins of Alzheimer's disease, stokes and brain aneursyms have been linked to GI track problems.[191]

As we get into the late 60s and early 70s of life, if not sooner, we can no longer digest certain foods as well as before. Foods high in protein may become more difficult to digest, and require longer GI tract transit times which correspondingly cause infrequent and hard to pass bowel movements and internal poisoning due to the blocked intestinal wastes. Even some whole plant foods may be difficult to digest with age.

For example, some people may no longer be able to consistently eat some kinds of high cellulose and insoluble fiber foods, such as lettuce and spinach, without constipation or having difficulty in passing stools. It means that the diet must be adjusted to eliminate these foods, or else eat them less frequently. Another example is nuts. I love eating nuts of all kinds, especially with frozen bananas (that is, frozen peeled bananas somewhat thawed), but now they cause me too much constipation, so I just enjoy my frozen bananas without the topping, which, to me, tastes like vanilla ice cream. In any case, the protocol is the same to avoid constipation: eliminate or lessen the frequency of eating such foods.

---

[191] https://www.theguardian.com/society/2023/aug/24/digestion-issues-could-be-warning-sign-of-parkin.

The Only Cure for Constipation

The simpler you eat on the food chain the more constipation-free you will be, both now and in the future.

"The adulterated, unnatural, false, man-made foods of present-day civilization are the underlying physiological causes of all evils which humans are prey – especially of all kinds of diseases. Health will not return, nor can it be regained through drug remedies or the various medical treatments, since supreme, absolute, paradisiacal health is ruled by the laws of diet!" - Professor Arnold Ehret, *Thus Speaketh the Stomach and the Tragedy of Nutrition*.

Constipation literally divides a life into two parts: when you have it and when you don't. The efforts at correcting the condition are more than compensated and rewarded by being relieved of the nagging problem and no longer having worries about getting more serious diseases.

Adopting a whole plant food diet and having little, if anything, to do with a meat and dairy based diet, which has been proven to damage human health beyond anyone's skepticism, including lowering the strength of the immune system and increasing one's risk of getting heart disease and stroke, is the best assurance that anyone can have against premature death due to disease.

Anyone who eats whole plant foods almost exclusively will have all the enzymes, nutrients and antioxidants the body needs to support a strong immune system, and need not fear getting gastrointestinal diseases, or pandemic diseases like COVID-19. And you can bet that these diseases will grow in kind and severity as we continue through the century.

To ensure that your immune system protects you from infectious organisms, take care of your gut microbiome by eating nutritious, whole foods, and stay away from foods and their combinations that cause constipation, diarrhea, gas and acidity which decrease the strength of the immune system.

"Eat to live, instead of live to eat." This was the dictum of Socrates, the most exemplary of the Greek philosophers. It represents the tried and tested way of health attained by the Greeks during the Golden Age of Athens. It is good advice for all of us.

It is said that growing old is the tragedy of life, as if there weren't enough tragedies already in everyone's life. Maybe it is true for some people, but I have found that the deterioration of flesh and bone that comes with age is just another challenge that needs to be addressed. While no longer young, and in no way having met all of the challenges of life, I feel confident, after having met and overcome some of them that other health issues can be dealt with in similar ways.

The upshot of the book is that no one has to be the tragic victim of a gastrointestinal disease, or any other disease, for one can avoid them.

"He who does not know food, how can he understand the diseases of man?" – Hippocrates.

Chapter 6 Alcohol and Constipation

Alcohol dehydrates the body because it causes the loss of bodily fluids. It can be severe at high altitudes, such as when flying across country in an airline, or if you happen to live in dry areas of the world. The more concentrated the alcohol, the worse the reaction will be. Plus, imbibing alcohol in excess can cause rejection by vomiting, which further dehydrates the body.

However, alcohol activates peristalsis, which, as discussed in Chapter 1, is the muscular action that sends food through the digestive system. Within hours of imbibing alcohol, waste elimination will be stimulated.[192]

So, the bad and the good can be working at the same time. The bad is the dehydration, causing waste material to become hard and dry as the body recovers lost electrolytes from the waste, and the good is that it stimulates waste elimination.

The bad can be remedied by drinking water whenever using alcohol. However, very few people ever do this or mix alcohol with water. The result for many, if not most people is that constipation worsens with alcohol use.

Each person must determine if, together with dietary change, their alcohol consumption should be cut back or remain as it is to cure themselves of constipation.

Perhaps the worst part about drinking alcohol is that it increases bodily acidity, which not only contributes to constipation but can lead to many other complications as described in this book.

---

[192] https://www.healthline.com/health/diarrhea-after-drinking-alcohol.

Chapter 7 Nocturia and Constipation

Nocturia is the need to urinate at night on a more frequent basis than normal. It is similar to incontinence, which is a sudden urge to urinate but you cannot hold the urine long enough to get to the toilet. Both can be caused by a weakening of the urethra muscles because of age.[193]

Nocturia is directly influenced by constipation because clogged up or backed up wastes can press against the urinary bladder and exert a force that pushes against the bladder, which can cause the bladder to send signals to the brain for it to be emptied before it is full, making a person urinate more frequently than normal at night, but also during the day as the same term ("nocturia") is typically used for both a daytime and night time bladder disfunction.

For most men, however, there is another difficulty – the walnut-sized prostate gland located between the bladder and penis. The duct or tube through which urine is expelled, called the urethra, passes through the prostate gland. Men with BPH (Benign Prostrate Hypertrophy) or other prostate dysfunctions, such as prostate cancer, can be so affected that they cannot urinate at all, requiring a trip to the hospital to have a catheter inserted into the bladder for relief. And it all begins with the symptom called nocturia.

But what you will not find discussed online or elsewhere in the literature is the simple fact that some people are just more active than others and have a higher metabolism, which enhances the ability of the body to more rapidly expel what it ingests.

---

[193] https://www.nia.nih.gov/health/urinary-incontinence-older-adults#:~:text=Urinary%20incontinence%20means%20a%20person,to%20avoid%20their%20normal%20activities.

Chapter 8 Proper Food Combinations

"Cook not, neither mix all things one with another, lest your bowels become as steaming bogs...for I tell you truly, if you mix together all sorts of food in your body, then the peace of your body will cease, and endless war will rage in you." - Attributed to Jesus in *The Essene Gospel of Peace, Book One.*

Most people eat combinations of foods, such as ientrées and side dishes, but combining certain foods can easily lead to stomach and intestinal troubles, unless you have what is called a cast-iron stomach, a term that describes people who seem to be able to eat all kinds of things without ever feeling ill. Only two examples are meat and potatoes (proteins combined with starches), and acidic fruit and sweet fruit. Before food can nourish the body, it must be digested, but each type of food requires different digestion gastric juices, with corresponding different digestion times.

As stated in the chapter on The Digestive System, digestion is a chemical process assisted by chewing that breaks down food into constituents that can be assimilated by the body.

Food combination laws are rules of nature that are based on the principle that different types of foods require different times for digestion, and cause the secretion in the stomach of different types of gastric juices, some being more acidic, some less acidic. If we eat foods that cause more alkaline (less acidic) gastric juices to be secreted for their digestion together with foods that require more acidic gastric juices for their digestion, the gastric juices combine and tend to null each other out, resulting in food in the stomach that is difficult to digest. This leads to a variety of complications, such as increased digestions times, stomachaches, headaches and fermentation, and, when the food passes through the intestines, putrefaction, gas and breeding of parasites.

When foods are difficult to digest, the energy reserves of the body are called into play to assist in the job of digestion. It should not be surprising that you feel tired after eating a big meal of improperly combined foods – the traditional nap after a Thanksgiving dinner.

The stomach does not decide what foods to put into it. It leaves that job to the brain. But when cultural norms and traditions and the memory of what we like to eat come into play, mistakes are made.

The Web adequately covers many aspects of proper food combining. A good website on proper food combining at the time of this writing is: https: //www.acidalkalinediet.net/correct-food-combining-principles.php.

However, some Web articles on food combining do not stand up to careful scrutiny. For example, some tell us that combining nuts with sweet fruits is an improper food combination. But based on my experience, and what nutritional experts tell us, fatty nuts (like walnuts and pecans) combine well with some sweet fruits, such as bananas. Other sweet fruits, such as apples that have a high-water content, can make the nuts indigestible.

In *The Sunfood Diet Success System*, David Wolfe explains that nuts are actually fat-dominant, not protein-dominant, foods because they consist mostly of fat. He explains that the fat in nuts and seeds allows the natural sugar in sweet fruit to be time-released, which helps digestion and provides more long-term energy. Combining sweet fruits with fatty nuts and seeds is an acceptable food combination, contrary to some of the articles on the Web.

The food combination laws should be learned, even if one or two of them are not correctly stated on the Web. The laws that are not correctly stated on the Web at least err on the safe side so that by observing them you will not be hurting yourself. Set goals for yourself to rigidly put the laws into practice.

The rules of food combining are soundly rooted in physiology and thoroughly tested by experience.

"More than sixty years spent in feeding the well and the sick, the weak and the strong, the old and the young, have demonstrated that a change to correctly combined meals is followed by an immediate improvement in health as a consequence of lightening the load the digestive organs have to carry, thus assuring better digestion." - Herbert M. Shelton, *Food Combining Made Easy*.

I enjoy many foods by themselves, but I'm an inveterate mixer. I prefer to combine foods rather than practice a mono-diet, but perhaps at the expense of maintaining optimum health.

I learned the food combination laws the hard way, by trial and error, and suffered all the stomachaches and other complications of improperly combining foods. Very probably, you will learn them the hard way too. It took me about a year to put all the laws into practice without making further mistakes.

Five of the food combination laws that are important on any diet, including a whole plant food diet, are as follows.

1. Don't Eat Proteins with Starches

Examples: Meat (a protein food) and potatoes (a starchy food); also, nuts (a protein and fat food) with mangoes or dates (starchy foods).

2. Don't Eat Starches with Acid Fruit

Example: Potatoes or peas (both starchy foods) eaten with tomatoes (acid fruit).

Note that tomatoes combine well with leafy greens and fatty plant foods like avocados.

3. Don't Eat Starches with Sweet or Sub-Acid Fruit

Example: Beans or peas (starchy foods) added to green smoothies that contain sweet or sub-acid fruit.

I have my own rule for this – don't add vegetables other than leafy greens to green smoothies. I've had too many stomachaches from breaking this law, so I make it easier to remember by excluding all vegetables (except greens) from my green smoothies that contain sweet fruit.

4. Don't Eat Sweet Fruit with Acid Fruit

Example: Pineapple (an acid fruit) eaten with bananas or dates (sweet fruit).

Note that sweet fruit combines well with sub-acid fruits, such as apricots.

5. Don't Eat Proteins with Sweet Fruit

Example: Nuts (a protein food) with dates (sweet fruit). Higher protein foods, such as spirulina, are even worse combinations with sweet fruit, and they cause severe gas resulting from the fermentation that occurs, and constipation. Bananas are an exception because they combine well with nuts and seeds.

The above food combination laws cover some of the errors typically made on a whole plant food diet. Additional food combination laws should also be learned. As explained previously, you can learn about them on the Web.

Digestion Times and Food Combination Laws

To aid in preparing meals, the digestion times for different foods should also be learned. Obviously, if we combine foods that require completely different digestion times, we're asking for trouble. Digestion times for different foods are adequately covered on the Web.

Typically, digestion times and proper food combinations go hand in hand. For example, as stated in the chapter on The Digestive System, it takes 6-8 hours for just the stomach to digest a pizza, and the digestion time for the grease and fat in a hamburger can go beyond three days.[194] [195]

When the food combination and digestion time laws are obeyed, digestion is greatly improved and overall well-being is enhanced. When they are broken, stomachaches, headaches, excessive flatulence, constipation or other complications can and do result,

---

[194] https://kauveryhospital.com/blog/lifestyle/how-long-does-it-take-to-digest-a-pizza/.
[195] https://www.sciencealert.com/here-s-what-eating-a-big-mac-does-to-your-body-in-an-hour.

which can quickly turn what started out to be a good day into a bad one.

"Improved digestion results in general improvement in all the functions of life. Many and great are the benefits to flow from improved digestion." - Dr. Herbert M. Shelton, *Food Combining Made Easy*.

How to Determine the Starch Content of Foods

Food labels (Nutrition Facts Labels) typically give the amount of total carbohydrates, sugar and fiber, but not the amount of starch in the food. The starch content might be published on the Web, but if it's not, here's how to determine the starch content of any food from its Nutrition Facts Label.[196]

From the food label on the product package, or as given on the Web, get the weights in grams of total carbohydrates, sugars and fiber and plug them into the following equation:

Starch = Carbs − (Sugars + Fiber).

Example 1: Carrots. Per the Web, a 61g serving of carrots has 6g carbs, 2.9g sugars and 1.7g fiber.

Starch (g) = 6g − (2.9g + 1.7g) = 6g − 4.8g = 1.2g

1.2g/61g = 2%

Carrots are 2% starch. Since the starch content of carrots is very low, it is a non-starchy vegetable.

---

[196] https://www.csidcares.org/treatment/reading-food-labels/#:~:

The Only Cure for Constipation

Many articles on the Web differ on whether carrots are starchy or non-starchy vegetables. Some articles say carrots are starchy vegetables while others say they are non-starchy vegetables. This is another example of conflicting information found on the Web.

Example 2: Beets. Per the Web, a 100g serving of beets has 10g carbs, 7g sugars and 2.8g fiber.

Similar to the above computations, beets are 0.2% starch. It is a non-starchy vegetable.

Example 3: Turnips. Per the Web, a 122g serving of turnips has 8g carbs, 4.6g sugars and 2.2g fiber.

Similar to the above computations, turnips are 0.1% starch. It is a non-starchy vegetable.

Example 4: Cinnamon. Per the Web, a 7.8g serving of cinnamon has: 6g carbs, 4.1g sugars and 0.2g fiber.

Similar to the above computations, cinnamon is 21% starch. Cinnamon is a starchy food. It should not be used with protein foods or with sweet or sub-acid fruits.

If you learn not to eat foods that do not go well together, you will have smoother and more frequent bowel movements.

As the proper combination of hydrocarbons in your vehicle's fuel determines how it runs, so your life will run smoothly if your foods are eaten in their proper combinations. In my opinion, if positive feedback is not received by the body in one or two days on any food that is eaten, no matter what the type or variety – fruit, vegetable, Superfood, herb or any other kind of food – then that

The Only Cure for Constipation

food should either be eaten in a more ripe condition, in smaller quantities, in proper combinations with other foods, or it should be avoided completely. The body is no fool. It recognizes foods that disagree with it or do it harm by giving us warning signals. Our job then is to correctly interpret these signals.

Chapter 9 The Best Medicine

"He is the best physician that knows the worthlessness of the most medicines." - Benjamin Franklin.

Alternative medicine practitioners tell us that practically every aliment of which humans are prone can be effectively prevented or controlled through lifestyle changes. Depending on the health issue and the person, it may take a combination of medication and lifestyle changes, but no matter what route is taken, lifestyle changes must be included. This chapter will show why I believe lifestyle changes are the most important.

A principle of naturopathic healing is to provide the body, through the proper foods, nutrients and other essentials it needs for health. A healthy diet can remedy a multitude of health issues, ranging from nutritional deficiency to constipation, and from general fatigue to diseases of the vital organs of the body. Nutritionists tell us that a healthy diet is the single most important lifestyle change a person can make for health.

But what do we see? Everywhere we look, foods are being sold that are harmful to health.

A typical example as seen in food stores and supermarkets across the country is regular or wholewheat bread, which can be anything from the real thing to one of the many spongy, artificially-colored and artificially-flavored chemicalized varieties with aspartate or MSG (both flavor enhancers), L-cysteine (a conditioner), malto-dextrin (a thickener), diacetyl tartaric acid ester of monoglycerides (DATEM), sodium stearoyl lactylate (SSL), mono- and diglycerides, monoglyceride derivatives, lecithin, and polyglycerol esters of fatty acids (PGEF) which are all emulsifiers, and a host of other synthetic chemicals added for ease of processing and other commercial purposes. One has only to read about these additives to realize the damage they can do to the human organism.

The ancient Roman caution, "Caveat Emptor" ("Let the Buyer Beware"), carries the same weight and significance today as it did in the days of the Roman Empire.

People of every age, gender, nationality and ethnic group have benefitted from simple but important lifestyle changes, the same changes that most likely were ignored or neglected in their lives previously. More and more people are realizing that it is in their best interests to take care of their bodies. After all, it is not our doctor's, spouse's, friends' or the Government's responsibility to attend to our health, it is our responsibility. The Government cannot do it for you. To be sure, you have to do it yourself.

It has been repeatedly proven that a healthy lifestyle is more effective than drugs or medical intervention, such as hospitalization and surgery, in treating any disease, and constipation is no exception.

A good example is Robert E. Kowalski, who ate the Standard American Diet (S.A.D.) for years before suffering a heart attack at age 35, followed by multiple bypass surgeries, and who took blood pressure mediation for years thereafter, but who discovered that most of the medication he was prescribed could be dropped by making some simple but important lifestyle changes. He later wrote a book about it.[197]

Many doctors have not been trained in nonpharmacological

---

[197] Robert E. Kowalski, The Blood Pressure Cure; 8 weeks to Lower Blood Pressure Without Prescription Drugs.

disease management. In addition, few people are familiar it. But it is the most effective way to remedy or control practically any health issue. Some of the nonpharmacological things that can be done for health can literally transform a person into a vibrant, healthy and brand new creation, free of sickness and disease.

The information now available in the human health field, and particularly in the science of foods and nutrition, can be put into practice to greatly reduce a person's chances of being afflicted by almost any disease. The importance of adopting a diet that avoids refined and processed foods, high cholesterol foods, trans fats and omega 6 vegetable oils, with their dire effects on human health, cannot be denied, and continues to be the number one behavioral change for health in general, regardless of the health issue, but particularly for a constipated condition or high blood pressure.

Next in importance is exercise. Then weight control. In fact, just about anything that is proven conducive to health can be included in an effective constipation management program, regardless of the particulars about an individual's condition and the time he or she may have spent on medication.

Perhaps the leading factor in the effectiveness of lifestyle changes for health and longevity is the level of commitment of those who embrace them. If a person is convinced that health is in their best interests to maintain and protect, and they make it a top priority in their lives, and are convinced that true health is best attained by their own efforts, then their level of commitment is likely to be high and they will have the best chances of curing themselves of whatever ails them.

"Always bear in mind that your own resolution to succeed is more important than any other thing." - Abraham Lincoln.

The Only Cure for Constipation

The best way to be convinced that health is best attained by one's own efforts is to read about foods and nutrition, especially the books written by well-respected nutritionists and nutrition-minded medical doctors, such as Nathan Pritikin, Dr. Michael Greger, Dr. Caldwell Esselstyn, Jr., T. Colin Campbell, Dr. Ann Wigmore, Arnold Ehert and Norman W. Walker.[198]

If the attainment of genuine health required no knowledge or effort or discernment whatsoever on the part of people, then everyone would be remarkably healthy. But even if you are only half-hearted about lifestyle changes and don't stick with them for very long, you still stand to benefit from the experience of having tried them.

The following lifestyle changes for true health are endorsed in addition to medication by many mainstream medical doctors and other health care professionals, but they are endorsed *without* medication by well-respected alternative medical practitioners such as those cited and footnoted above, and also by many online sources such as those cited here.[199] [200] [201] [202]

1. Dietary change. A change in diet is the most recommended lifestyle change for reversing and healing a medical condition. Why? Because of what has already been explained about the

---

[198] Dr. Michael Greger, How Not to Die, T. Colin Campbell, The China Study, Dr. Caldwell Esselstyn, Jr., Prevent and Reverse Heart Disease, Dr. Ann Wigmore, Be Your Own Doctor, Arnold Ehret, The Mucusless Diet Healing System, Norman W. Walker, Become Younger.
[199] https://www.mayoclinic.org/diseases-conditions/high-blood-pressure/in-depth/high-blood-pressure/art-20046974.
[200] https://www.heart.org/en/health-topics/high-blood-pressure/changes-you-can-make-to-manage-high-blood-pressure.
[201] https://www.healthline.com/health/high-blood-pressure-hypertension/lower-it-fast.
[202] https://www.medicalnewstoday.com/articles/318716.

The Only Cure for Constipation

causes of disease, that they are principally diet related. It is by far the best solution that anyone can incorporate for safeguarding their health and healing a disease or other health issue.

People in this country should be the healthiest people on earth. It certainly seems that way since there are now more varieties of health promoting and sustaining foods available to us than ever before, and many of them are organically grown.[203] But we are not the healthiest people because of our preferences for artificial, man-made foods and drinks, our giving way to cultural norms and traditions about foods, and our unwillingness, and even refusal, to abide by Nature's laws that govern health and well-being.

"We must close our ears and our minds to the false prophets posing as "experts," who ignorantly recommend "man-made foods" that are slowly but surely hastening our end." - Professor Arnold Ehret, *Thus Speaketh the Stomach and the Tragedy of Nutrition.*

"Among the many thousands of species of creatures living on the earth, only humans and some of their domesticated animals (dogs, cats) try to live without food enzymes. And only these transgressors of nature's laws are penalized with defective health." - Dr. Edward Howell, *Enzyme Nutrition.*

Whole plant foods are different in many ways from other foods. Apples, when planted in the soil, produce additional apple trees. Raw nuts planted in the ground produce other nut trees. Even a harvested potato when planted yields at least another potato plant. But many of the foods that are consumed on ordinary diets

---

[203] Organically grown produce does not have the highly toxic herbicides and pesticides that are sprayed on conventionally-grown crops, and it is not grown in mineral-starved soils which are used to produce conventional crops.

have been devitalized by heat treatment. Cooking destroys the life force properties that are in whole plant foods. Plant a cooked bean or tomato or a roasted nut in the ground and it will not grow. Cooked foods, including refined and processed foods, do not promote or sustain health, but are harmful to the body.

The best diet is the one that meets the energy and nutrient needs of the body and produces the least negative effects. If one of these negative effects is evident, then one or more of the foods eaten should be avoided, and all you have to do is find out which ones. For most people, it means a diet consisting of a large volume of fresh, raw fruits and vegetables to meet the body's nutrient and energy needs, with perhaps some concentrated foods, such as nuts and seeds included.

Just as exercise must be tailored to the person, so it is with foods.

2. Daily exercise. Exercising moderately for 30 minutes a day is extremely important for health in general, and can lower a high blood pressure condition by 5 to 8 mm Hg. And whatever is good for health in general helps the entire system because all parts of the body are interconnected. Long walks, cycling, swimming and lifting weights helps not just one or two parts of the body, but all parts. One needn't worry about exercising temporarily raising blood pressure, which occurs during exercising, since it lowers blood pressure on an average basis. Also, the time it takes to recover from an increased heart rate during exercise decreases as one becomes more fit. Exercise is essential for regular bowel movements, since one of the things that leads to constipation is physical inactivity.

"People who are physically fit recover quickly from exercise. Their pulse rates and heart rates return to baseline much faster that those who are less fit." - Carol Tavris, *Anger, the Misunderstood Emotion.*

3. Weight Loss. It is well known that weight gain affects a person's susceptibly to getting disease. It is also well known that weight gain increases blood pressure and that weight loss lowers blood pressure. Some reports tell us that blood pressure may be reduced by 1 mm Hg for every 2.2 pounds (1 kilogram) of weight lost.[204]

Ask anyone who has lost a lot of weight, such as a hundred pounds or more, how they did it and they will likely reply with pithy statements such as: "eat less and move more" and "throw out the steer and cow."

4. Detoxification

The topic is discussed in detail in the next chapter.

5. Stress reduction. Stress raises blood pressure. Medication is widely prescribed and taken for nervous conditions, but no drug can cure nervous disorders. You can cope with stress through medication, but you can't get rid of it that way.

The best way to handle stress is through rest and relaxation, doing the things that Nature compels us to do, but which we never seem to find the time to do. The remedy is so simple that it is generally overlooked, but it is true.

Chronic stressors include repeatedly spending time with people you dislike, working for someone you dislike, and experiencing

---

[204] https://www.mayoclinic.org/diseases-conditions/prehypertension/diagnosis-treatment/drc-20376708.

road rage. Avoiding such things, or getting away from other things that cause stress levels to spike, lowers blood pressure and promotes overall health and longevity.

Another form of stress is noise. Noise is unwanted sound, and its effect on people differs from person to person, but any noise that is upsetting to where it arouses anger will raise blood pressure, and if prolonged will cause chronic stress. Like other stressors, noises are best avoided wherever possible.

Prayer and meditation are known to relieve stress, bitterness, anger, disappointment, heartbreak, old grudges and frustration, all of which contribute to bowel disfunctions like constipation, and other maladies such as high blood pressure. Both practices have a cathartic effect on the mind.

Independent clinical studies have shown that *meditation* (not medication) lowers blood pressure significantly. Researchers have found that regularly practicing techniques like Transcendental Meditation helps in numerous ways. Consistent practice can lower systolic pressure by more than 10 mm Hg and diastolic pressure by more than 6 mm Hg.[205]

If it were not for taking these "time outs" from daily struggles, we would be swamped and continually irked by the many stresses that are daily imposed on us. But when we practice prayer or meditation, a profound peace descends upon us. It leads not only to the momentary relief of worry and stress, but to improved mental health and emotional stability. It relieves us of the oppressive urgency of the present, the regret of the past and the fear of the future.

---

[205] S.H. Shepherd, How to Cure High Blood Pressure.

The Only Cure for Constipation

6. Stop smoking. If you smoke, stop. Cold turkey is perhaps the best way. It's how I stopped after smoking 2-3 packs per day for over 30 years when I became convinced that it was doing me irreparable harm. Smoking reduces the oxygen available to the lungs, replacing it by carbon monoxide, carbon dioxide, and cancer-causing chemicals that are sprayed on the tobacco leaves during their growth, and, if paper cigarettes are used, cancer-causing chemicals are sprayed on the cigarette paper, and all these things cause lung cancer and heart attacks.

It is said that if anyone ate a pack of cigarettes (20 cigarettes), it would kill them.

It has been the experience of many in the natural health field, and my own experience as well, that making the effort required to put healthy lifestyle changes to work brings about closure not only to health issues like high blood pressure,[206] arthritis[207] and constipation, but also dispels health worries about getting other diseases.

Furthermore, the sense of accomplishment and the boost in self-esteem that follows being able to heal yourself of a health issue are priceless rewards.

---

[206] Ibid.
[207] For a detailed discussion of the causes of, and the cure for, arthritis, see the book, S.H. Shepherd, The Cure for Arthritis.

Chapter 10 Detoxification

Detoxification is the normal, ongoing and automatic bodily process that removes accumulated toxins (poisons) from the body to make the tissues and organs function properly. But when the toxins build up to where the normal process cannot keep up with them, it predisposes a person to sickness and disease, and requires additional measures for their removal. These additional measures are purgation through natural food cleansing, and fasting, and they are what most people mean when they use the term detoxification.

Toxins accumulate in the organs and tissues of the body from eating animal-based foods, cooked and starchy foods, and refined and processed foods. A lifetime of eating these foods necessitates purgation before the body can be restored to health.

The body also receives toxins from the environment, for example, from exhaust fumes, pesticides and municipal drinking water. The body tries to purge them all, but when it contains more poisons than it can handle, the result is ill health. However, when the body is cleansed of its toxins and is daily given living plant foods, health reigns.

As stated previously, constipation is a major cause of internal toxicity due to the rapid growth of parasites that thrive and flourish in rotting intestinal wastes. Stopped up wastes are a fertile breeding ground for many kinds of non-friendly parasites, including tapeworms which can cause many complications. A person may have a bowel movement once a day and think that everything is fine, but everything is not fine.

Detoxification is the rite of passage everyone must go through to become genuinely healthy. Internal cleansing is required before rejuvenation and health can be achieved.

Toxic wastes continue to build up until corrective action is taken. To avoid suffering from toxic waste health disorders, the most important thing we can do is to reduce or eliminate the intake of foods and supplements that cause the toxic waste buildup, and eat whole (raw) plant foods instead. Antioxidant-rich foods are known to stop or even reverse toxic buildup. Whole plant foods are high in antioxidants that neutralize the poisons and help to flush them out of the system.

Fasting

Fasting assists the body's self-cleansing process which helps us attain optimum health. When the body is sufficiently cleansed of the poisonous waste materials that have accumulated from years of wrong eating, then comes true health, health as you may have never experienced it before. We need to use fasting, as well as colonics and enemas, to purify our bodies of the filth that has accumulated in them from years of wrong eating. Fasting is discussed in detail in the book, *A Christian Diet*, which is listed in the Bibliography. More will be said about colonics and enemas later in the book.

Fruit and Vegetable Cleansing

Whole plant foods possess the highest level of nutrients found in any food, and bestow numerous health benefits, some of which are yet to be discussed in this book. An abundance of vitality is available to anyone who adopts a whole plant food diet. When toxins are removed from the body through the self-cleansing process that is enhanced by eating raw plant foods, you feel great.

The Only Cure for Constipation

Detoxification really takes off when raw plant foods are consumed exclusively. If you are on an ordinary diet, the detoxification process is, for all practical purposes, ineffectual because ordinary diets cause toxic wastes to build up to the extent where thorough detoxification is not possible.

To purge the body of its accumulated toxins, stop eating all meats, cheeses, grain products like breads, and other foods that are known to be harmful to the body, such as refined and processed foods, and eat only foods that the body thrives on for health, which are whole plant foods such as vegetables and fruits. Eat very little, if any, cooked foods during the detoxification process.

David Wolfe in his book, *The Sunfood Diet Success System*, states that detoxification stops when cooked foods are eaten. The dangers associated with cooked foods, why they are detrimental to human health, are described in the chapter on Dangers to Avoid.

We need to take detoxification into stride when we start eating whole plant foods exclusively. Continue through the healing process trusting that the body is gaining health by what it is doing. Know that drugs that block these symptoms also block the detox process.

<u>Transient Discomforts</u>

What is known as "toxic overload" may occur when the detoxification/self-cleansing process is ramped into high gear by a sudden shift to an all whole plant food diet.

The sudden shift causes an abundance of toxins to be released into the bloodstream all at once, and, as confirmed by many raw food eaters and nutritional experts, this may cause flu or disease

The Only Cure for Constipation

like symptoms to occur creating discomfort and malaise. People have gotten seriously ill from transitioning too quickly to a whole plant food diet. This is why a gradual transition to whole plant foods exclusively during detox is recommended. The purpose of eating some cooked foods during the transition period is to slow down the detoxification process in order to avoid toxic overload.

Living plant foods are so powerful that they immediately start cleansing the body of its poisons. Their life force actions on the body drive out toxic wastes into the bloodstream for their elimination through the normal elimination organs of the body (including the skin). The powers of living plant foods are clearly evidenced by the signs the body gives when it detoxifies itself on these foods.

Wastes released into the system from eating a whole plant food diet initially make you feel unhealthy, and during the self-cleansing process you may experience some signs of ill health. But this is natural and normal. It is caused by the toxins within the tissues and organs of the body being released into the bloodstream. Feelings of fatigue, dizziness, and the signs cited below may be experienced until the "house cleaning" is completed. But when the toxins are eliminated, the feeling of true health is experienced.

The possible ill effects of detoxification should not in any way dissuade the reader from proceeding with a whole plant food diet, since it is the way to true health. They are provided so that you will not be surprised by them when you undergo detoxification.

The following things are normal and last only during the detoxification process.

Normal signs of detoxification: frequent urinations and/or bowel movements, diarrhea, headaches, runny nose, colds, expectoration, loss of energy, feelings of melancholy, needing more sleep, etc., all indications that the body is purging itself of toxins. Additional signs of detoxification are found in Robert Morse's book, *The Detox Miracle Sourcebook*.

The transient discomforts of detoxification cause some people to quit a whole plant food diet before the benefits are obtained because they do not understand the detoxification process. But those who stick with the process experience the tremendous boost in vitality that follows self-cleansing, when the accumulated poisons are removed from the system.

"There is only one true healing modality – detoxification. It will bring the body's chemistry back into homeostasis (balance) and remove the toxic metals, elements and substances that don't belong there." - Robert Morse, N.D., *The Detox Miracle Sourcebook*.

Those who have never experienced detoxification cannot know what it is like. You can read about it in books, like this one, and in articles on the Web, but unless you have personally gone through it you will never know what it is like.

"A pure raw plant diet assists the body's cleansing efforts in the most natural way by eliminating any toxicity from entering the system and by simultaneously moving toxicity through the lymph and blood and out the body through the eliminating organs (the bowels, kidneys, liver, skin, sinuses and lungs). A purification of the diet enforces a self-healing and radical whole-body rejuvenation." - David Wolfe, *The Sunfood Diet Success System*.

In my opinion, the chief importance of detoxification is to relieve the body of the burden of all forms of constipation and peel away the coating of paste-like plaque formed on the walls of the

The Only Cure for Constipation

intestines after years of eating wrong foods, foods that are detrimental to health (this is discussed the chapter on Dangers to Avoid).

One of the things I learned during my first year on the whole food diet that was not covered in the books listed in the Bibliography, was that improper, or bad, food combinations can cause not only stomachache, headache, heartburn, and flatulence, but also constipation. Therefore, watch your food combinations during the detox process.

"It can be strongly said that the health of an individual is largely determined by the ability of the body to detoxify." - Joseph Pizzorono, N. D., and Michael Murray, N. D., *Encyclopedia of Natural Health*.

Chapter 11 The Causes of Disease

"The doctor of the future will give no medicines, but will interest his patients in the care of the human frame, in diet, and in the causes and prevention of disease." - Thomas Edison.

Diseases seem to wait in ambush, ready to strike and slay. But what are they really, at least according to our best scientific understanding, and what does this understanding tell us about how diseases may be cured? This chapter explores these topics.

Health issues uncommon in the past are frequently experienced today. Widespread and serious illnesses and diseases strike everyone, everywhere. How many people do you know who are suffering from a health affliction or disorder? How many readers of this book have heart disease or some other health issue they're wrestling with?

There are, no doubt, hundreds of diseases that afflict humankind, including all the fevers, tumors and contagion of human life. It is not the purpose of this book to chronicle all human diseases or to give an account of the known causes of them, but to explore some of the attempts made by man to understand, control and cure the diseases that beset him. Two views of diseases will be presented, the view commonly held by the mainstream medical profession, and the view held by modern nutritionists.

Bear in mind that since human diseases appear to have certain causes, and we have evidence that there are methods by which they can be avoided, there must be ways to cure them.

The Only Cure for Constipation

Mainstream Medicine View

The deadliest diseases in this country, and the most feared, are heart disease; cancer of the organs, including colon, bladder, lung and breast cancer, kidney disease, COVID-19, and the neurological diseases, including Alzheimer's disease and Parkinson's disease. According to mainstream medicine, the causes of these diseases are primarily foreign substances, including but not limited to bacteria, viruses and poisons that get into, or invade, the body.

The theory of infection is built around microorganisms; in short, microbiology, a product of laboratory work based on the proposition that microorganisms, which include bacteria and viruses, are responsible for the majority of our diseases. The attempts made by mainstream medicine to cure diseases are primarily efforts that are aimed at eradicating the foreign substances and organisms that are believed to cause the diseases.

The methods used by mainstream medicine to treat diseases include pharmaceutical drugs, antibiotics such as penicillin and erythromycin, and medical intervention such as hospitalization and surgery. Of course, vaccines are also used. Many of the drugs must be improved yearly by medical laboratories to counteract the proliferation of drug-resistant organisms that result from their use. Radiation therapy and chemotherapy are also used. These methods are, for the most part, all that mainstream medicine has in its arsenal against diseases.

As stated in the chapter on Standard Treatments for Constipation, standard medical treatments focus on achieving health through drugs. For headaches, take Aspirin or a similar product; for stomachaches or heartburn, take antacids; for infections, take antibiotics; for constipation, take laxatives; for cancer, take chemotherapy or radiation therapy. But even considering drugs like penicillin which can halt the spread of a disease, drugs do not possess the ability to cure, and there are risks associated with all drugs. Also, drugs have been known to lodge in the system for decades after their use.[208]

Diseases which are today considered eradicated, such as malaria, smallpox and poliomyelitis, are not eradicated in the true sense of the word, because the viruses or parasites associated with them still exist. They are merely prevented from causing excessive harm through vaccination, which is the most common form of immunization used against diseases.

There are, of course, exceptions. Leprosy and inflammation of the eyes (uveitis, a disease that can cause blindness), can both be cured through drug therapy as long as sanitary measures are also put in place, unless, in the case of eye inflammation, the cause is an autoimmune disorder. Both diseases were the scourge of the Middle East 200 years ago when many of the population suffered terribly from them. Physical blindness today is often prevented merely through sanitary measures.

Permanent cures of diseases by mainstream medicine are rare.[209] It is believed that many of the cures that are attributed to

---

[208] From the book, Prof. Arnold Ehret's Mucusless Diet Healing System: Annotated, Revised, and Edited by Prof. Spira.

[209] For example, the average cure rate for all types of cancer by mainstream medicine, except for skin cancer, is 17% per G. Edmond Griffin's book, World Without Cancer. It is believed to be more like 6% per Rich Anderson's book, Cleanse & Purify Thyself. A 2019 American Cancer Society Web article states that most cancers cannot be cured, but some can be controlled for months or even years. A cancer.net article sponsored by the American Society of Clinical Oncology (ASCO) states that chronic cancer is cancer that cannot be cured.

mainstream medical treatments would have occurred naturally without them.

Viruses and bacteria are everywhere and exist in everyone, but before they can proliferate and thrive in the body, they must have suitable soil. Nutritionists believe that it is the waste material in the body that affords the germs the suitable soil for them to proliferate and produce the symptoms of disease.[210]

The Nutritionist View

Nutritional experts do not believe that "germs" or bacteria and viruses are the primary causes of disease. Rather, it is the presence of undigested and uneliminated rotting food waste accumulated over time in the tissues and organs of the body due to eating wrong kinds of foods and overeating. In their view, these things mean that elimination of the foul material is the only rational means of curing disease.

To put it another way, they believe that disease is the result of intestinal occlusion, the clogging up of food wastes in the large intestine (colon), and that correcting the situation through proper diet is the only way that the body can rid itself of disease, recover and then resume a life of health.

They believe that disease symptoms are manifested as a result of this poisoning, and that they are signs the body gives when it attempts to eliminate the poisons. Malaise and fatigue are two typical signs of internal poisoning, and so are sores and rashes.

---

[210] Louis Pasteur (1822-1895) gave the world the germ theory of disease, but he was never able to prove it. On his death bed he stated, "the germ is nothing, the terrain is everything." In other words, the soil of the body is far more important than any pathogens that attempt to invade it.

In other words, disease is an attempt to rid the organism of the foul material with which it is contaminated. Also, disease symptoms are the outward manifestation of an automatic internal bodily cleansing process. For example, nausea and fever result from the body's natural attempts to rid itself of morbid, toxic material that has accumulated in the tissues. They may be triggered by, but they are not caused by, "infectious organisms" that invade the body.

What do nutritionists say is the answer?

"In food lies 99.99% of the causes of all disease and imperfect health of any kind. Consequently, all healing, all therapeutics will continue to fail as long as they refuse to place the most important stress on diet." - Arnold Ehret, *Mucusless Diet Healing System*.

The cure for disease, then, is not to treat the symptoms, including the pains that may result from the disease, but the underlying causes of the symptoms.

"The foods you consume can heal you faster and more profoundly than the most expensive prescription drugs, and more dramatically than the most extreme surgical interventions, with only positive side effects. They can prevent cancer, heart disease, Type 2 diabetes, stroke, macular degeneration, migraines, erectile dysfunction, and arthritis – and that's only the short list." - T. Colin Campbell and Howard Jacobson, *Whole, Rethinking the Science of Nutrition*.

Many of the diseases that afflict us appear to be the result of either an unwitting ignorance of the unalterable laws of nature, or a willful refusal to abide by these laws. Adopting a whole plant food diet and restricting food intake to manageable amounts of the most easily digestible foods helps to ensure that every seed of sickness is extirpated from the body.

"Man's health or his disease of every description, directly result from food intake. His state of mind may be a contributing factor, but the fall of mankind in the final analysis is "sin of diet." The real physiological cause of all evils, especially the physical ailments of mankind can be traced directly to the present day accepted diet of civilization." - Arnold Ehret, *Rational Fasting and Roads to Health and Happiness*.

An old saying is:

One quarter of what you eat keeps you alive. The other quarter keeps your doctor alive.

Many medical researchers and nutritionists claim that the primary cause of most human diseases are the foods that are commonly consumed, and that it is the consumption of these foods that leads to the life-shortening diseases of heart disease, cancer, diabetes and the neurological diseases. It is my belief that this claim will be proven to everyone's satisfaction in the years to come, impacting many popular beliefs regarding age-related health issues. An example is the degenerative disease of arthritis, which many nutritionists, including Dr. Ann Wigmore, believe is caused by harmful dietary practices.

"Healing is no accident. All nature heals itself when causes are removed and the conditions of health supplied." - Dr. Herbert M. Shelton.

It has been my experience and observation that we are more than capable of causing our own sicknesses. We unwittingly bring sickness and disease upon ourselves through dietary practices that are contrary to the laws of nature. The body requires a variety of nutrients to keep itself in health, but seldom finds them in the foods that are commonly eaten. It requires enzymes for proper digestion, but they are destroyed by heat, and almost all refined and processed foods are heat treated. Deprived of the nutrients and other essentials it needs to enhance the body's self-cleansing process, the natural law of cause and effect determines the outcome, which is ill health.

According to nutritional experts, local treatments are harmful to the entire body, not just the part or parts that may be displaying the symptoms. They contend that almost all attempts made by mainstream medicine to cure diseases are not successful in a true sense, but can, at best, only forestall the diseases from taking over and killing the patients in the short term.

Healing does not come from drugs. It comes from natural bodily processes, such as self-cleansing, or detoxification, that remove accumulated toxins, obstructions and acidosis from the body, from rest, and from providing the body with the nourishment it needs.

The beacon of warning, the clarion call for proper action, has been sent out. We need to become more our own doctors than ever before, and the sooner it starts the better it will be for us, to avoid the unnecessary suffering associated with medical treatments that are not designed to heal.

Medications can temporarily relieve pains and inhibit inflammation, but they can weaken the immune system, and are often habit forming. Many published medical books and articles available to us about human diseases reveal that patients must often cope with the toxicity of the substances that are prescribed for their illness as well as the illness itself.

The Only Cure for Constipation

As powerful as the medical profession is, it seems to have eyes that cannot see and ears that cannot hear in its quest for cures for diseases. Because of this, we are in danger of being continually affected in adverse ways by medical treatments as time goes by.

As emphasized throughout this book, when confronted with a health issue, we should do everything in our power to resolve it without resorting to doctors. When the cause and effect relationship between a health issue and what we are doing to ourselves becomes apparent to us, sknown, as well as the proper steps that are needed to put the solution into effect.

Furthermore, as evidenced in hospitals throughout the world, many patients of chronic and acute diseases die despite the treatments they receive, or even because of them. In 2014, in the United States and Europe, prescription drugs were the third leading cause of death, after heart disease and cancer. In 2016, a John Hopkins University study indicated that the third leading cause of death in this country was medical errors.[211] [212]

As discussed in detail in the book, *Don't Take the Shots* referenced in the Bibliography, we now have evidence that many of the lives lost to COVID-19 were lost needlessly and avoidably to vaccines and inaccurate medical diagnosis.

These things have led many people to seek second or even third opinions about their health issues. Blind faith in the medical profession has eroded since earlier days, but many are not finding suitable alternatives, nor have they gained sufficient knowledge

---

[211] https://pubmed.ncbi.nlm.nih.gov/25355584/.
[212] https.//www.vekluryhop.com/important-safety-information/?gclid=Cj0KCQjwqhttps://www.hopkinsmedicine.org/news/medicine.org/news/media/releases/study_suggests.

about foods and nutrition to convince themselves that dietary change is necessary and the need to take charge of their own health is paramount.

Mainstream medicine spends billions of dollars of federal, state and private funds each year trying to find cures for diseases, especially COVID-19 and the nominal top 10 deadliest diseases in this country. But cures for these diseases remain elusive.

Despite continuing assurances from medical research labs that cures are in the offing (which, by the way, has been going on for quite some time, especially for the top 10 diseases), it is doubtful whether cures will be realized as long as the underlying causes of diseases are believed to be foreign substances or organisms.

Therefore, as previously stated, to effectively deal with any disease, the underlying cause, or causes, of the disease must be known. Mainstream medicine's attempts at curing diseases have not met with success in the vast majority of cases, including COVID-19 and the top t0 leading causes of death in this country, which strongly suggests that the causes that are commonly attributed to diseases are not really the underlying causes at all, but only contributing causes or factors that can localize a disease to certain parts of the body.

It appears that disease will remain, at least for the present, somewhat of a mystery to mainstream medicine, maybe as much of a mystery as disease was to the "medicine man" of yesteryear. Having directed its energies and skills primarily at the suppression of the symptoms of diseases, mainstream medicine appears to have missed the mark.

Without a sufficient knowledge about foods and nutrition we

remain wholly ignorant of how to achieve optimum health. The knowledge needed is best obtained by reading books and utilizing other learning tools, such as the Web, to discover the truth about these vital subjects. Furthermore, I believe it is the key to recovering from a disease and preventing disease from taking root in the human soil of the body in the first place.

"Get Wisdom! Get understanding!" - Prov. 4:5.

Mucus-forming Foods

Professor Arnold Ehret, a nutritionist popular in Germany in the early 1900s and later in America, was probably the first to recognize that mucus-forming foods cause waste obstruction in the body, and that the obstruction causes disease. In his book, *The Cause and Cure of Human Illness*, he states that there are two main reasons for human disease: 1) constipation caused by mucus-producing foods, and 2) overeating, i.e., eating more than is necessary, more than the system actually needs – more calories than the body needs.

Mucusless foods are non-starchy foods. They include raw fruits, leafy greens and non-starchy vegetables.

Ehret healed himself of Bright's disease (a kidney disease), and cured many hopeless cases of chronic diseases by putting his patients on his mucusless diet and fasting regimen. Many of the patients were very serious cases with terminal diseases, and lay on their deathbeds. Many had gone through other therapies, including those requiring strict diets, but without success. He also cured those who suffered from degenerative diseases, both acute and chronic. After following his mucusless diet for only a short time, all of his patients regained their health. Can conventional medicine, with its use of pharmaceutical drugs and/or medical intervention, including surgery and chemotherapy that are intended to cure diseases, make such claims?

Ehret believed that the buildup of mucus in the body was the first and foremost cause of disease, and that health can only be restored when the buildup is removed from the body. He did not claim that mucus was the only cause of every disease, but that it was the main cause present in almost all diseases.

"There is no man in existence in western civilization whose body has not been continually stuffed since childhood with cow milk, meat and eggs, potatoes and cereal products." - Arnold Ehret, *Mucusless Diet Healing System*.

In his landmark book, *The Mucusless Diet Healing System*, first published in 1922, Ehret released to the world his incredible findings regarding a starch-free diet consisting of raw fresh fruits, leafy greens and non-starchy vegetables (mucusless foods) which he claimed was the optimal diet for human health. The book is considered by many nutritionists to be the definitive work on the prevention and curing of human disease through diet and fasting.

Ehret's book has become one of the most important texts in the modern raw food movement. Raw food eaters have repeatedly confirmed that the mucusless diet heals diseases.

As revealed in many of the books that are listed in the Bibliography, it is the firm conviction of many nutritionists that starchy foods, which are mucus-producing foods, cause human disease. The reason for this is explained in the chapter on Dangers to Avoid.

The body attempts to rid itself of mucus through the lymphatic system which typically results in various forms of expulsion or expectoration, such as excessive saliva, clearing of the throat, coughing, sneezing, colds, flus, and congestion of the lungs, throat and ears. Nutritionists believe that these are all signs of excessive mucus in the body.

"All disease is finally, nothing else but a clogging up of the smallest blood vessels, the capillaries, by mucus." - Arnold Ehret, *Rational Fasting and Roads to Health and Happiness*.

Berg's Tables, which appear in Appendix I, list what foods are acid-binding and acid-forming. These terms are synonymous with mucus-binding and mucus-forming, respectively. The most mucus-producing foods are meat and grain products, whereas fruits and vegetables are the most mucus-binding foods.

When the large intestine, or colon, becomes obstructed, it hinders the absorption of nutrients in the body. Poor nutrient absorption leads to nutrient deficiency. If the food is nutrient-deficient in the first place, then even less nutrients are assimilated by the body.

If true, then we live in a very sick world, a world in which almost everyone is addicted to mucus-producing cooked and starchy foods, with their devitalizing properties and adverse effects on heath.

Again, Professor Ehret:

"Disease is an effort of the body to eliminate waste, mucus and toxemias, and the system assists nature in the most perfect and natural way. Not the disease but the body is to be healed, it must be cleansed, freed from waste and foreign matter, from mucus and toxemias accumulated since childhood. You cannot buy health in a bottle, you cannot heal your body, that is, cleanse your system, in a few days, you must make "compensation" for the wrong you have done your body all during your life." - Arnold Ehret, *Mucusless Diet Healing System*.

According to nutritionist Robert Morse, mucus-forming foods are responsible for many types of inflammation in the body, such as the diseases that end in "itis", including bursitis and arthritis.

A Slightly Different View of Diseases

Some nutritionists believe that diseases are best explained as the result of three causes. The first two are brought about by the practice of consuming foods and drinks that are harmful to the body, or the practice of combining foods improperly. The third is what some consider to be a possible cause of diseases.

1. Toxicity

2. Acidity

3. Heredity / Genes

Let's examine each.

Toxicity

Toxicity is internal poisoning that is brought about by accumulated waste material in the body. According to nutritionists, it is the most common ill health condition prevalent today. It is mainly the result of eating the wrong foods, such as animal-based foods that are baked or deep-fried in oils; starchy foods, including doughnuts, sweet rolls, pasta and bread; and other refined and processed, heat-treated foods, including canned, jarred and most packaged snack foods. Toxicity results from the morbid accumulation of toxins and food wastes in the organs and tissues of the body, and is similar to mucus buildup from eating mucus-producing foods.

Secondary causes of toxicity of the body include the ingestion of chemical preservatives and man-made additives that are found in refined and processed foods, and the ingestion of pesticide residues on foods. Common medical practices also cause toxicity of the body, such as vaccinations and prescription drugs.

Poisons can also get into the body from the environment, from municipal drinking water, car exhaust fumes, cigarette smoke, and toxic chemicals that we become exposed to in the home and on the job. All contribute to the toxicity of the body. Some of these pollutants are carcinogenic or mutagenic. It seems very likely that exposure to these toxic substances will continue for some time to come in our society.

The result is that the body is made toxic by substances it ingests or is exposed to. The good news is that certain foods, such as green leafy vegetables, protect us from the harmful effects of carcinogens like no drug can. Chlorophyll in green plants detoxifies the liver and bloodstream and neutralizes environmental pollutants. To receive this protection, all we need to do is include greens in our diet.

Many people take inorganic substances in the form of multivitamin/mineral supplements on a daily basis. Billions of dollars are spent each year in America alone on these substances. Also, many take medication every day as prescribed by their doctors. Inorganic substances and drugs are not properly utilized by the body but are treated by the body as toxins. Many of them get stored in the body's tissues.

Some of the internal damage caused by toxic substances heals automatically. But when overloaded with toxins, the body cannot eliminate the poisons fast enough, which causes them to accumulate in the tissues. And that is when they can cause harm, such as weakening the immune system.

Commonly consumed foods, including meat, fish, eggs, and dairy products, contain substances that are toxic or otherwise harmful to the body, including carcinogens, hormones, dioxins, bacteria, and other contaminants that can accumulate in your body and remain there for years. Every year we hear of meat products contaminated with E. coli, listeria, campylobacter, or other dangerous bacteria that live in the intestinal tracts, flesh, and feces of animals.

Other commonly consumed food products contain substances that are known to be harmful to human health, including table salt, refined sugar, hydrogenated oils, preservatives, artificial colors and sweeteners, excitotoxins, such as monosodium glutamate (MSG), and GMO (Genetically Modified Organism) food products such as High Fructose Corn Syrup (HFCS). All are unnatural substances produced by man-made processes.

We should avoid as much as possible all of that "crapola."

Evidence from X-rays and autopsies of people with long histories of poor eating habits, such as eating a lot of cooked and starchy foods, reveals a plaster-like coating formed on the inner surfaces of the large intestine, or colon. This coating, or what many investigators call "plaque", prevents foods from being fully digested and assimilated, and often causes obstruction of the colon. In time, the coating builds up to where the intestines become mostly or even totally obstructed. A thorough discussion of intestinal obstruction, with sketches, is found in Dr. Norman W. Walker's book, *Become Younger.*

The Only Cure for Constipation

The colon is the septic tank of the body. It needs to be cleaned out periodically for health. But if this is not attended to, and foods which are harmful to the body continue to be eaten, toxification of the entire organism is the result causing not only cancers but many types of serious health disorders such as stroke. The consensus of many modern nutritionists, including those whose books are listed in the Bibliography, is that internal poisoning and morbidity are precursors of illness and disease.

Self-cleansing or detoxification, as explained in the chapter on Detoxification, is what removes accumulated toxins from the body.

Constipation is a major cause of internal toxicity. It is worsened by the rapid growth of parasites that thrive and flourish in the rotting intestinal wastes. Stopped up wastes are a fertile breeding ground for many kinds of non-friendly parasites, including tapeworms which can cause many complications. A person may have a bowel movement once a day and think that everything is fine, but everything is not fine, for a single bowel movement a day is a sign of a serious health concern. It is a warning signal given by the body that something is wrong and should be corrected as soon as possible. Foods that are devoid of fiber, such as meats, dairy and white flour products, are known to cause such constipation.

When in good health, one can expect to have at least as many bowel movements per day as meals taken per day. It is not only based on my own experience, but is common to strict vegans and raw vegans who have learned what foods to avoid and what are proper food combinations. It is one of the gauges used for telling whether a person is in good health. Real freedom, no matter where you may be living, is constipated-free eliminations, probably the best comfort you can ever have.

The Only Cure for Constipation

Toxic wastes continue to build up until corrective action is taken. To avoid suffering from toxic waste health disorders, the most important thing we can do is to reduce or eliminate the intake of foods and supplements that cause the toxic waste buildup, and eat raw plant foods instead. Antioxidant-rich foods are known to stop or even reverse toxic buildup. Whole plant foods are high in antioxidants that neutralize the poisons and help to flush them out of the system.

As stated previously, "A pure raw plant diet assists the body's cleansing efforts in the most natural way by eliminating any toxicity from entering the system and by simultaneously moving toxicity through the lymph and blood and out the body through the eliminating organs (the bowels, kidneys, liver, skin, sinuses and lungs). A purification of the diet enforces a self-healing and radical whole-body rejuvenation." - David Wolfe, *The Sunfood Diet Success System*.

Acidity

Acidity is a blood condition mainly brought on by eating too many acid-forming foods. When we eat foods typical of a cooked meat and/or pasteurized milk diet, which are acidic foods, the blood becomes thick and heavy which causes clogging in the tissues and is known to adversely affect the arteries and lymphatic system, and cause poor circulation and elevated blood pressure.

According to leading nutritionists, acid-forming foods are responsible for many of the diseases and health issues and that are prevalent in the world today, including diabetes and kidney disease.

When we eat whole plant foods such as raw fruits, vegetables and leafy greens, the blood's condition becomes normal, which is alkaline, and is not thickened which results in improved circulation and reduced blood pressure.

Acidity in the body also occurs when foods are combined incorrectly. Foods improperly combined inhibit digestion and cause discomforts such as stomachache, abdominal pain, constipation and fermentation and gas, the resulting putrefaction of which causes bodily acidity and produces toxins that pollute the blood (bodily toxicity). Constipation, in turn, leads to more acidity and toxicity of the body, a vicious spiral that can cause many other complications including serious diseases.

Acid-forming foods include foods high in protein, such as eggs and beans as well as meat and dairy products. Even ingesting a single meal high in meat, dairy and grain products (such as bread, pasta and rice), can cause, in a few days or weeks depending on the food, hard passage of wastes. High protein foods cause the nutrients to stick together, which leads to cellular starvation and death. The foods also cause mucus production in the body, which is considered a forerunner of disease.

Refined grain and cereal products, refined sugar, meat products, including sausages and hot dogs of beef or pork, and pasteurized dairy products are widely eaten today. All leave behind a residue of toxic acids in the body. Modern refining techniques, including the use of high-temperature heat treatment and over-cooking, destroy the alkaline mineral salts found in natural foods that act to neutralize these acids.

If the acids go unchecked, they form hard acid deposits in the system. The soft tissues of the body, including those in the throat and anus, are the first affected. Eventually, the acids are deposited in the muscles, joints and ligaments of the body, which can cause arthritis and many other diseases such as bursitis, colitis and diverticulitis.[213]

Cooked foods create acidity in the body, whereas uncooked (raw) plant foods alkalize the body.

"People are becoming more and more acid. The public is not told this because the powers that be do not want people to know what is being done to them. In the last few decades, this fatal condition appears to be on the increase." - Rich Anderson, *Cleanse & Purify Thyself.*

Homeostasis is the tendency of the body to maintain itself in stable chemical equilibrium. It is the process whereby the body tries to balance or stabilize itself from an acidic condition to a normal alkaline condition.[214] Obviously, the effectiveness of the body's ability at doing this is encumbered or enhanced by the foods that are eaten.

An acidic blood condition often results from a nutrient deficient diet, such as the standard American diet. The reason it is nutrient deficient is explained below. If the diet is continued, the blood condition worsens to where the body's attempts at homeostasis are not sufficient in neutralizing the acids. Toxic acids the body cannot expel as waste in its on-going self-cleansing efforts are stored in the tissues and joints which can lead to diseases. Vegetables, including leafy greens, carrots, cabbage, tomatoes, raw nuts and seeds, are alkalizing to the body, creating an alkaline blood condition that is conducive to healing and regeneration.

---

[213] Margaret Hills, Treating Arthritis: The Drug-Free Way.
[214] Robert Morse, N.D., The Detox Miracle Sourcebook.

The Only Cure for Constipation

Refined and processed foods have been heat treated (cooked) and almost always contain refined salt (table salt), refined and processed ingredients such as high fructose corn syrup (HFCS) and monosodium glutamate (MSG), and man-made flavors, colors and preservatives, none of which are natural products.

Americans eat more cooked food than any people on earth, and spend more money on doctor bills and healthcare than any people on earth. It appears to be more than a coincidence. The fast food franchises, as well as other eating establishments, grill, fry, bake, steam-heat their foods, or use dehydrated foods that have already been refined and processed using these methods. It has been known for years that these methods destroy important food components such as enzymes, vitamins and other nutrients, and alter the chemical properties of the foods.

In contrast, nutritionists tell us that our bodies are biologically suited for alkaline-forming foods, which are the fruits and vegetables found in nature. Since these foods neutralize acids that can cause disease, heartburn, upset stomach, indigestion, flatulence and other complications, we need to eat plenty of these foods.

Stress produces acidity in the body. High levels of stress have been linked to all kinds of physical and mental disorders. This acid-producer seems to have taken up permanent residence in our society.

"You must remove the obstructions and acidosis, if you don't, the cause remains as you have treated only the effect which can be swelling, pain or other symptoms. These are nothing more than natural defenses of the body in response to the cause. De-toxification is the only logical answer that will yield a lasting cure.

The Only Cure for Constipation

Alkalization is the method by which detoxification starts. Alkalization neutralizes acidosis. Detoxification not only alkalizes the body, but also gives the body the added energy it needs to clean itself." - Robert Morse, N.D., *The Detox Miracle Sourcebook*.

Berg's Tables, in Appendix I, list what foods are "acid-forming" and "acid-binding." According to these tables, meat and grain products are the most acid-forming foods, whereas fruits and vegetables are the most acid-binding foods.

Whenever we eat animal products, a particularly harmful acid is produced – uric acid. Animal protein is complex protein that must be broken down before it can be assimilated by the body. The breaking down process results in the generation of an excessive amount of uric acid. Since the muscles of the body have an affinity for uric acid, it is initially deposited in the muscles. When the saturation point is reached and uric acid is sent to the kidneys, uric acid crystals are formed which can cause kidney stones and gout. According to Norman W. Walker's book, *Become Younger*, uric acid crystals can cause arthritis.

After about 8 to 10 hours inside the stomach, undigested proteins start to rot. The exceptionally poisonous byproducts of rotting causes an excess loss of fluids and electrolytes, and often provokes vomiting.[215]

Nutritionists tell us that if we ate nothing but raw fruits and vegetables, our blood would be alkaline most of the time, except for periods of undue stress or when other causes of blood acidity are introduced.

---

[215] https://www.gutsense.org/constipation/alcohol.html.

The chapter on the Blood describes how blood tests are used in medical diagnosis in assessing the acidity of the body.

Heredity / Genes

Gregor Mendel, an Augustinian friar who lived in the 1800s in what is now the Czech Republic, is the founder of the science of genetics. He discovered dominant and recessive traits, and that parents can hand down a trait that is unlike themselves. He showed that a trait can be hidden for many generations and then become evident in offspring. Hence, scientists believe that people may have a proclivity for certain diseases because of their genetic makeup.

Scientists after Mendel have used his discoveries to help explain diseases that are believed to have a genetic basis. For example, it is believed that thin blood vessels of forefathers can have an effect on the lives of their offspring.

According to the National Human Genome Research Institute (NHGRI), an institute of the National Institutes of Health (NIH), genetic disorders are diseases caused by changes in the DNA due to mutations or damage to chromosomes.

Sickle cell anemia, a condition in which there are not enough healthy red blood cells to carry adequate oxygen throughout the body, is considered by the NHGRI to be an inherited disease. The reasons for this appear to be based on earlier work by scientists, such as Linus Pauling and Janet Watson on the molecular bases for sickle cell disease, which established the inheritance pattern of the disorder and of monogenic diseases in general, and later from a wide variety of experimental studies on mice involving DNA vectors and the development of gene delivery systems. The problem I see with this research is that it appears to assume rather than prove the conclusion that the disease is inherited. If you start off assuming a conclusion, you operate in a closed system.

The medical industry receives much of its funding for medical research from the NIH, which is part of the US Department of Health and Natural Resources. Many of the findings and positions of the Institute are based on the results of this research. It is speculative whether all the positions taken by the NIH, or for that matter the NHGRI, reflect views other than those of the medical industry. This is not to say that their findings should be dismissed, but that they should be viewed in a proper perspective.

Most scientists agree that certain physical characteristics, such as eye color and hair color, are inherited. But other characteristics, such as left-handedness, appear to have no biological basis. Hand preference, for example, is believed to arise as part of the developmental process that differentiates the right and left sides of the body (called right-left asymmetry) which occurs at an early age.

Scientists have often speculated that certain disorders, such as mental aberrations or psychiatric disturbances, may have a biological or inherited basis. However, there appears to be no scientific proof or evidence of these things. It is now believed that environmental factors may contribute to such disturbances.

Some researchers say that genetic variations confer only a small risk of disease. The redoubtable Hereward Carrington in his book, *Vitality, Fasting and Nutrition*, observed that whenever disease, which he believed was the penalty of broken natural laws, is ascribed to heredity, we escape from taking responsibility for that disease. He preferred to ascribe diseases to being due to the simple fact that like causes produce like effects.

The Only Cure for Constipation

Heredity does not mean that we will get the diseases of our forefathers, even if we knew what they were, which most of us do not. It only means that we could get their diseases if, in fact, they were caused by genes, which is yet to be proven based on my researching.

The subject of inherited diseases is a controversial one. But despite the amount of detailed and extensive work that has been done by the medical profession on diseases, there has been very little, if any, scientific proof that any disease is caused by genetic deficiencies in DNA. Some diseases appear to have a biological basis, but the hard evidence is lacking to show they are the result of genes. There appears to be no consensus, either among modern medical researchers or nutritionists, that diseases that are ascribed to heredity are actually based on genetics. This may change in the future, but it appears to be the situation at the time of this writing.

"What you eat every day is a far more powerful determinant of your health than your DNA or most of the nasty chemicals lurking in your environment." - T. Colin Campbell and Howard Jacobson, *Whole, Rethinking the Science of Nutrition*.

Since we are helped or harmed by any experience in life, a lot depends on our reactions to what happens to us. Nowhere is this more important than in dealing with health issues. We can take a doctors' advice and rely on medication for our health issues, hoping that the doctor knows best how it should be managed, or we can learn how to take care of ourselves. One of the premises of this book is that anyone can eliminate constipation and avoid numerous other health issues simply by putting into practice the insight and knowledge gained about foods and nutrition.

The Only Cure for Constipation

"Life is like a game of chess. To win you have to make a move. Knowing which move to make comes with insight and knowledge, and by learning the lessons that are accumulated along the way."
- Author Allan Rufus.

Why do natural cures work better than standard medical treatments? As stated previously, the reason is because they are not designed to treat the symptoms, including the pains that may result from the disease, but the underlying causes of the symptoms. Furthermore, mainstream medicine places emphasis on treating specific, localized symptoms. Modern drugs are prescribed to correct one symptom or another without effectively strengthening the overall state of health. But the body is an integral organism consisting of many parts, with every part connected with every other part. All parts of the body receive the same blood and lymphatic fluid supply to support its needs. No one part can be diseased and the rest be healthy. Similarly, when one or more parts of the body are healed of ill health, the other parts of the body benefit as well.

One may wonder, as I have, why we do not all get diseases, such as polio, diphtheria, typhoid or cholera. The answer from a nutritionist's viewpoint is that there is no suitable soil in our bodies in which these diseases can take root. It appears to be the only reason we do not all get diseases. Microorganisms cannot harm us as long as our organism functions in a normal, healthy way. Microbes such as viruses are harmless if the body's defensive mechanisms, including the immune system, are in good working order. A weakened immune system can be caused by drugs, improper diet, unhealthy lifestyles, health issues such as obesity, advanced age, diabetes, lung disease and heart disease, and these things can put people at increased risk for COVID-19 and its variants.[216] [217] [218] [219]

What if You Already Have a Disease?

According to nutritional experts, if a person already has a disease but deprives the microorganisms their food and renders the human soil unsuitable for their growth, then the disease can be cured. From this perspective, there is hope that disease may not only be prevented, but cured through natural means.

Disease should not be looked on as an affliction brought on by fate or Providence, but something primarily, or perhaps even solely, brought on by an ignorance of the unalterable laws of nature, and most notably the laws governing foods and nutrition.

If fasting can cure almost all diseases of which the human race is susceptible, and it appears that it can,[220] then what does it tell us about how diseases and other health disorders originate? Doesn't it clearly reveal that the principal cause of almost all human maladies lies in the foods that are eaten? Does it not assuredly implicate improper diet as the main cause of our many ailments?

The body's ability to fight illnesses is determined by the health of the immune system. As stated in Appendix III, Bacteria in the Gut,

---

[216] https://www.hopkinsmedicine.org/health/conditions-and-diseases/coronavirus/coronavirus-the-covid19-vaccine-and-epilepsy.
[217] https://www.cdc.gov/coronavirus/2019-ncov/need-extra-precautions/people-with-medical-conditions.html.
[218] https://katv.com › news › local › high-blood-pressure-d.
[219] For a discussion of the immune system and the COVID-19 virus, see S. H. Shepherd, Don't Take the Shots.
[220] A detailed discussion of fasting is given in S. H. Shepherd, A Christian Diet.

70-80% of the cells of the immune system reside in the gut.[221] The gut microbiota aid in food digestion and fight off invading microorganisms. Certain diseases, such as cancer, repress the immune system and allow increased attacks by unfriendly microbes and viruses. Nutritionists tell us that the best way to improve the health of the immune system is to eat whole plant foods.

"A whole food plant-based diet deals with so many diseases and conditions that you begin to wonder if there isn't just one basic disease cause – poor nutrition – that manifests through thousands of different symptoms…Poor nutrition causes vastly more diseases than the disease care system currently acknowledges; but good nutrition, in contrast, is a cure for all those diseases and more." - T. Colin Campbell and Howard Jacobson, *Whole, Rethinking the Science of Nutrition.*

I have never seen, but would like to see, the statistics on those who have contracted the COVID virus and those who have adopted a whole plant food diet and having little, if anything, to do with consuming meat and dairy products, which have been proven to damage health, including lowering the strength of the immune system. Assuming a correct diagnosis and not one that is really the flu (as was the case with so many of the COVID-19 cases), I would venture to guess that the statistics would be very low indeed.

Chapter Summary

People get diseases for a reason. Mainstream medicine attributes

---

[221] https://pubmed.ncbi.nlm.nih.gov/33803407/.

the causes of disease primarily to foreign substances, including but not limited to bacteria, viruses and poisons that get into, or invade, the body.

From a nutritionist standpoint, however, disease is primarily a consequence of something that is wrong with the diet, the particulars of which may differ from person to person, but it is always a prime factor. The principal causes of the diseases of humankind are: 1) a weakening of the immune system that causes unfriendly bacteria to proliferate inordinately in the waste material and 2) the blood poisoning by the toxins that are thereby produced; and it is all because of the foods that are commonly eaten.

Disease symptoms occur as a result of the body attempting to rid itself of the poisons.

When the cause and effect relationship between a disease and what we are doing to ourselves becomes apparent to us, then the best solution will be known, as well as the proper steps that are needed to put the solution into effect.

Improvements in health of practically any kind can be said to start when the vital roles of foods and nutrition in human health are fully realized. The knowledge gained, and the practical know-how to implement the knowledge, allows diseases such as constipation to be cured, which, in the case of constipation, minimizes the threat of getting more serious diseases.

It is no coincidence that urgent care centers in this country have become as numerous and widespread as fast-food restaurants.

Chapter 12 The Cure for Constipation

To cure constipation, something must be changed, and that something should be obvious by now. The most important change is diet. It means ending old eating habits by not giving in to food cravings that are harmful to the body, and learning new food choices and proper food combinations.

The cure depends on being attentive to the signs that the body gives in the ways that have been described, letting us know what is good for it versus what the mind often tells us is good for it. The protocol is to put health before satisfying cravings for certain foods, and replace taste appeal with health appeal.

For example, we may be convinced that we need to eat certain foods because we were raised on them, or because they're popularly advertised, or simply because we like them, even though they cause constipation. The type of change we are talking about involves learning about foods and their effects on constipation, and eating foods that do not cause the problem, effectively removing constipation from the equation.

The lifestyle changes described in the chapter on The Best Medicine are recommended, with minor exceptions as seen below. The changes may be done together or one at a time, but the more that are done the better, for they work cumulatively and synergistically to end constipation.

1) Dietary change
2) Exercise
3) Weight Loss
4) Detoxification (required whenever there have been years of eating foods that are harmful to the body)

The Only Cure for Constipation

5) Stress reduction

Most of the above items are recommend for a constipated condition by health care professionals when they prescribe medication.

If you're already having 2-3 defecations per day, then there may be no need for Item 3 (detox). But for most people, all five Items are required.

Many books and articles published on the Web, and also many practicing physicians, recommend cessation of smoking as part of any positive lifestyle change. I agree that it is a positive change for health, and that if it has not already been done then certainly it should be done, but I do not include it in the cure because it adds little in comparison to the other changes.

As discussed previously, exercise is essential for regular bowel movements since one of the things that leads to constipation is physical inactivity. The reason for including stress reduction is because it can induce a person to binge or overindulge on foods that cause constipation, such as refined and processed snack foods, candies, pastries and ice cream.

If you are slim and already work out daily, then you may exclude Items 2 (Exercise) and 3 (Weight loss), which leaves: dietary change, detoxification and stress reduction to be incorporated. Otherwise, I recommend all five items be done and get to where you are working on them concurrently.

We are highly conditioned in our culture to seek quick fixes for whatever goes wrong, from automobile tire repair to health issues, and standard medical treatments for most diseases and health disorders, including constipation, rely heavily on achieving health

The Only Cure for Constipation

through drugs. But there are no quick fixes for constipation, because one of the facts about it is that it takes at least 2-3 days to see any improvement from any of the positive lifestyle changes which, together with the availability of affordable drugs, causes many people to give up trying to cure themselves.

Health improvements typically take time. Nature is not on the 9:15 PM express to the suburbs. She does not rush, but takes her time as necessary to complete her work. The damage done to the system by years of unintentional wrong eating requires correction by the body's self-cleansing process before improvements are noticeable.

To reach the goal, do not stop until the changes are working. It means not quitting when you get frustrated, which assuredly will happen. For some people, it requires a matter of weeks to lose their constipation. For others it takes longer. It all depends on the level of commitment and the history of the disease.

Be careful what you eat. Monitor your progress by keeping a record of everything eaten daily, in the morning, afternoon and evening, and particularly the foods that you know from your self-education are causing the problems. Jot down the foods that you remove from the diet, noting the day and the time of day, and, after 3-5 days, see what effect it has on your condition. If you don't write them down, you will lose track and not remember what foods were excluded or eaten at what times.

Continue with the program and review your notes every 3 or 4 days until you have cured yourself of constipation. You learn all the while how to become your own doctor. The result is fewer doctor visits and doctor bills. It means saving money that would have been spent on drugs, not to mention having to suffer the side effects of the drugs.

The Only Cure for Constipation

You learn what foods and lifestyle changes work best for you by trial and error, guided by logic and commonsense.

Remember that GI tract food transit time, the time it takes for food to travel from the mouth to toilet, varies from individual to individual, and this is especially true during the transition period of the cure, which is the time it takes from starting the cure to when its positive effects are seen. It becomes shorter and reaches the optimum of about 2 to 3 days (48-72 hours) when you are constipation-free. That does not mean that you will have a bowel movement every 2-3 days, but that it takes 2-3 days for food to complete its transit from the mouth to the toilet.

When you are eating foods that do not cause constipation, the frequency of bowel movements per day typically will be the same as how many meals are eaten per day, which for most people means 4-5 or more bowel movements per day.

A simple way to determine the food (GI tract) transit time is by eating two or three servings of corn on the cob, frozen kernel corn, or canned corn, assuming that you do not eat them at every meal. Write down when they were eaten and watch for the undigested corn kernels to be expelled in the toilet. The intervening time is *your food transit time*, regardless of whether you are constipation-free.

As stated previously, for healthy, unconstipated people, who do not eat oils, meat, dairy or bread products, it is normal to have at least three bowel movements *per day*,[222] or one about every 8 hours. But since we tend to eat large meals and it usually takes 2-3 or more defecations to expel the wastes of a single meal, *for a healthy person it is normal to have a bowel movement every 4 or*

---

[222] Elizabeth Lipski, Ph.D., CCN, Digestive Wellness.

The Only Cure for Constipation

5 hours. Unconstipated stools are soft and free flowing, and do not require straining, and, they are typically on time.

There will be inner struggles with cravings that you will have to overcome, and times when you will backslide into your old ways of eating. After all, it is only human nature to vary what is eaten. But when you give in to an old craving while on the cure, you'll be able to see once their consequences, and you will become more aware of how old cravings cause constipation and harm the body.

If you focus on the goal you will get there, and learn a lot in the process. Again, the key thing to remember is "health appeal over taste appeal" while all the time enjoying every morsel. If something you eat goes well with you, then accept it, if it doesn't, reject it.

For inspiration, search and read the literature on the foods that you eat, checking details such as the starch content and how acid-forming they are, for this will confirm your decisions on the foods that should be avoided. It may also confirm your suspicions that not everything discussed online is correct. The information provided in subsequent chapters will assist you in making the right decisions, or see the books that are referenced in the Bibliography.

"Get Wisdom! Get understanding!" - Prov. 4:5.

If you're aware a particular food is acid-forming, either from experience (causes constipation, gas, etc.)[223] or from checking reputable sources such as Berg's Tables in Appendix I of this

---

[223] It is not always possible to tell acidity from taste alone; e.g., raw onions may taste bitter or acidic but they are acid-binding foods (Berg's Tables) and do not cause constipation for most people.

book, then you should curtail or eliminate it from your diet. An example is chocolate. Who doesn't like chocolate? It appears to be a fact of life that the foods we like the most end up causing the worst constipation, or harming the body in some other way. Chocolate is one of those foods, but beware that articles on the Web have different claims as to how it affects general health as well as GI tract health. For example, some websites claim that dark chocolate does not cause constipation but may speed up bowel movements, and that it is good for health because it has lots of minerals and fiber. Other articles say that its high fat content causes constipation.

The fact is, that chocolate is high in saturated fat, which causes constipation, and the caffeine in chocolate can cause dehydration which, as discussed previously, causes constipation. Nevertheless, how frequently you should eat chocolate, or any other food for that matter, or whether you should eat it at all, depends on how it affects your system.

Keep going until you are unconstipated. Bear in mind that no cure can be expected to work while eating habits are constantly counteracting the cure.

I am convinced that one of the keys to improving overall health and well-being is self-education about foods and nutrition. I believe it is the key to recovering from a disease, and preventing disease from taking root in the human soil of the body in the first place.

I believe that anyone who eats natural foods, foods that are low on the food chain, and puts health above gorging themselves on foods that are devoid of the life force nutrients and antioxidants that the body needs to maintain itself in health, is putting themselves at a high risk of getting a serious disease.

Chapter 13 Becoming Your Own Doctor

"The rest of the world lives to eat, but I eat to live." - Socrates (470-399 B.C.).

Several chapters have stressed the importance of diet change for health because of the strong ties that exist between the foods we eat and the body's natural ability to cure itself of constipation and heal and ward off other diseases. Emphasis has also been placed on the importance of taking charge of one's own health. More will be said about these strategic breakthroughs in this chapter.

No matter what age, gender or ethnic group, when a person starts eating healthy foods and learns how to properly combine foods, a doorway to health opens to them that may never shut again.

Numerous medical studies have attested to the fact that whole plant foods provide miraculous health benefits, and many books have been written about the incredible powers of raw plant foods to enable the body to cleanse itself of toxins and heal itself of diseases.

As you enter through the doorway to optimum health, you will find a marvelous and adventurous land verdant with resplendent gardens, orchards and colorful landscapes. The horizon stretches farther than the eye can see, and every day it rains at least once amidst plenty of sunshine.

As you take the exciting and rewarding journey into new realms of self-knowledge and self-awareness, you find that it enables you to become a more energetic and effective person, as a knowledge of foods and nutrition equips you to become your own doctor using the untainted and unaltered foods of Nature. This means fewer doctor bills and less time spent in the doctor's office.

For those who resort to the care of doctors or other health care professionals for whatever ails them, it is important to get used to the idea that you are, not just in the final analysis but now and during each and every day of your life, responsible for your own health. Since your body is the only one that you will ever have in this world, it only makes sense that health should be a top priority in your life.

It is our responsibility to take care of our bodies. It is not our doctor's, our spouse's, our friends' or the Government's. It is our responsibility. We should avoid foods that are harmful to health and eat foods that promote health and longevity. These are whole plant foods, replete with their life-giving properties. These are the foods that God and Nature intended for us to eat.

"But the foods which you eat from the abundant table of God give you strength and youth to your body, and you will never see disease. For the table of God fed Methuselah of old, and I tell you truly, if you live as he lived, then will the God of the living give you also long life upon the earth as was his." - Attributed to Jesus, *The Essene Gospel of Peace, Book One*.

Much of the joy, excitement and contentment we get out of life depends on how we take care of ourselves.

The quantity of food consumed during meals also matters for health. Nutritionists, such as Dr. Robert Morse, believe that digestive juices are secreted not in proportion to the amount of food eaten, but in proportion to the amount of food that is required by the system. (This may change your opinion about overeating.)

The Only Cure for Constipation

"The major characteristic of the diet of longevous people is low total calorie intake throughout life." - Dan Georgakas, *The Methuselah Factors*.

"The speed of elimination depends upon quantities and qualities of food and can therefore be controlled and regulated." - Arnold Ehret, *Prof. Arnold Ehret's Mucusless Diet Healing System: Annotated, Revised, and Edited by Prof. Spira*.

The body always lets us know how we are treating it. Understanding and heeding the warning signals the body provides helps us to maintain ourselves in concert with the laws of Nature.

This reveals a basic truth about our lives. The long-term consequences of our choices may be different than their immediate effects. To avoid the perils of constipation, one must not eat foods that cause it, notwithstanding the joy one may have in eating such foods.

We must examine our propensity to eat what is advertised and otherwise promoted by the many vested interests of the food industry, or that are dictated by cultural norms and traditions. Such foods are typically harmful to general health and GI tract health, so if we eat them, we must accept the consequences.

We must be concerned about the foods, the water and the air that we take into our bodies, and with the sleep and other forms of rest that we get, because they affect our chemistry and physiology for good or bad. Moreover, we must accept Nature's laws and stop trying to alter them to meet our own desires.

One would think that the mind would tell us exactly what to eat for mind and body health. But as everyone knows, that is not the case, for the mind is subtly influenced by many things, such as memories of past enjoyed meals and the price that was paid for them. As a result, most of the time our food choices are based on what we're most accustomed to eat, what is the most available and convenient and what is in keeping with cultural norms and traditions. In fact, unless the mind is sufficiently trained in the science of foods and nutrition, it is a rare exception indeed that foods that have health-appeal over than taste-appeal are ever considered.

The foods we put into our bodies every day play a much larger role in determining our health and well-being than many people are willing to accept. Some nutritionists say that it is the most important determinant of health. All other things, including exercise, fresh air, sunshine and rest and relaxation, are of lesser importance. However, moderate exercise and getting away from cramped quarters is very important, too, for all who live sedentary lives.

As stated in the chapter on The Causes of Disease:

"Healing is no accident. All nature heals itself when causes are removed and the conditions of health supplied." - Dr. Herbert M. Shelton.

It is commonly believed that foods are required for the body to produce energy and sustain health. However, there's a theory, called the vitality theory, endorsed by some nutritionists, that is based on the assertion that foods do not really energize us at all, but act only as stimulants.[224]

When animals get sick they instinctively abstain from all food.

---

[224] For more information about the vitality theory and the No Breakfast Plan, see S. H. Shepherd, A Christian Diet.

The Only Cure for Constipation

Can this be said of us? To a great extent, it cannot. Most people keep eating when they are sick on the mistaken belief that nourishment is needed for them to get well. Only rarely, such as in cases of acute fever, do we lose our appetite for food. Most doctors prescribe nourishment for those who are sick in hospitals, or who are otherwise under their care, and many patients force themselves to eat when the wisest thing to do would be to abstain from all food. It appears that in this context, animals are wiser than humans.

The healing powers of the body are fully at work when we live in concert with the laws of Nature, which means in part when we eat foods suitable for our biological makeup. But when we depart from Nature's laws by eating foods that do us harm, or do other things that are bad for health, such as depriving the body of adequate exercise, sunshine, fresh air and rest, we court disaster in the form of disease or some other troublesome health issue. If we understand the laws of Nature and abide by them, illness and disease are vanquished by the body's inherent life promoting and sustaining powers.

Nutritional experts and nutrition-minded doctors emphasize that sickness and disease cannot exist in a body that has cleansed itself of acidic and toxic wastes accumulated from years of wrong eating by the powers of living plant foods, the foods that are most conducive to human health, the foods that have the powers to heal. These foods allow us to trade our sorrows and disappointments for joy and gladness, and enable us to live simpler and less burdensome lives.

"Healthy food gives us the energy to be healthy and happy. When we eat food with energy, we become people with energy. The difference between people with energy and people without energy

The Only Cure for Constipation

is quire dramatic." - Sergei and Valya Boutenko, *Eating Without Heating.*

It was by learning about foods and nutrition that I was able to improve my health after suffering from many health issues for many years. I practice what I preach, and I believe that learning the truth versus hype about foods and nutrition is the key to reaching health goals. The insight and knowledge gained during the learning process is priceless, for very few things are as important as health.

Nobody is born with knowledge; it must be gained. When the knowledge required to promote and sustain health is gained and put into practice, practically any health issue that assails us can be effectively dealt with without the doctors' advice. It equips us to become, in many ways, our own doctors. This reality has far-reaching consequences for our health and well-being, providing numerous health benefits and preventing numerous health disorders.

"The excellence of knowledge is that wisdom gives life to those who have it." - Eccles. 7:12.

Some people like to be doctored, but it has never appealed to me unless I am truly ill. Because of the knowledge of foods and nutrition gained over the years, and having witnessed the healing powers of whole plant foods, I have learned not only that do I not need a doctor's advice on every little thing that goes wrong, but I can save myself a lot of time and money by curing my own health issues, and even more time and money by not getting many of diseases common to man.

Another reason for avoiding doctors is the widespread prevalence of medical malpractice cases due to clinical errors made by practicing physicians and their aids.[225] As stated previously in the chapter on The Causes of Disease, these things have led many people to seek second or even third opinions about their health issues.

No one really knows the state of their health better than each of us ourselves. And whether people realize it or not, most are seeking a healthier, less stressful, more simple, peaceful and harmonious life.

I'm glad that doctors are there when we really need them, like for accidents and traumatic injury, or when we have reached the end of our rope and nothing that we do works to correct the issue. But being your own doctor has advantages besides saving money on hospital stays and doctor bills. The sense of accomplishment and the boost in self-esteem that follows being able to heal yourself of a health issue are priceless rewards. Is there a doctor in the house? Yes, and it's you!

Being your own doctor in essence means learning all you can about foods and nutrition from informed sources, such as the books that are referenced in the Bibliography, putting into practice what you learn from these sources, and heeding the signals the body gives about what should and should not be eaten. You realize that the symptoms of any sickness are warnings that something needs to change about what you are doing. All the theory in the world does us no good unless we put it into practice.

"Life's greatest achievement is the continual remaking of yourself so that at last you know how to live." - Winfred Rhodes.

---

[225] NCBI defines medical malpractice as any act or omission by a physician during treatment of a patient that deviates from accepted norms of practice in the medical community and causes injury to the patient.

Chapter 14 Dangers to Avoid

This chapter explores some of the inherent dangers associated with the most commonly eaten foods, and why they should be avoided for a healthy and constipation-free life.

Meat and Dairy Products

Meats are high in proteins and fats but entirely devoid of fiber. Dairy products have less protein but as much as if not more fat than meats. Both are hard to digest, require long digestion times, and are the main causes of constipation in the Western world.[226] [227] [228] [229] There is more evidence that meat and dairy products cause disease than smoking causes lung cancer.[230]

Meat and dairy products are acid-forming foods, with high raking scores as seen in Berg's Tables in Appendix I.

Meat and dairy products cause high cholesterol in the bloodstream, which is the most common cause of high blood pressure, and a common risk factor for heart disease.

Cholesterol is a waxy substance found in the blood and most of the tissues of the body. It is produced in the liver through the

---

[226] https://shawellnessclinic.com/en/shamagazine/food-and-constipation-what-impact-does-milk-have/.
[227] Dr. Michael Greger, How Not To Die,
[228] https://www.webmd.com/digestive-disorders/ss/worst-foods-for-constipation.
[229] https://www.everydayhealth.com/constipation-pictures/foods-to-avoid-for-constipation-relief.aspx.
[230] Dr. Joel Fuhrman, Eat to Live: The Amazing Nutrient Rich Program for Fast and Sustained Weight Loss.

digestion of foods, and is necessary for healthy bodily functions, including cellular construction and hormone production. It is carried through the blood by lipoproteins, two of which types are high-density lipoprotein (HDL) and low-density lipoprotein (LDL), also known as the "good" and "bad" types of cholesterol, respectively.

Saturated fats and trans fats in the diet raise LDL (bad) cholesterol levels and cause the formation of fatty deposits in the arteries. The deposits harden, causing the arteries to become narrowed and also often choked with cholesterol plaque and calcium, which causes atherosclerosis. High blood pressure is caused by the hardened deposits forcing the heart to work harder to pump blood through the arteries. The more LDL in the bloodstream, the greater the risk of heart attack and stroke.[231] [232] [233]

Grains and Legumes

Grains are starchy and acid-forming foods. Their high acid-forming scores are seen in Berg's Tables in Appendix I. Starch is gooey and pasty. It is used for glues and hanging wallpaper. It sticks to the walls of the lower intestine and causes all kinds of problems, as discussed in the chapter on The Causes of Disease, and in this chapter in the section on Starchy Foods.

Legumes include peas, beans, peanuts and lentils. Legumes are commonly considered to be vegetables. Like grains, they are starchy foods, and for that reason I no longer eat them, with the

---

[231] https://www.heart.org/en/health-topics/cholesterol/prevention-and-treatment-of-high-cholesterol-hyperlipidemia/the-skinny-on-fats.
[232] https://www.mayoclinic.org › syc-20350800.
[233] https://www.cdc.gov/cholesterol/ldl_hdl.htm#:~:text=LDL%20(lo.

exception of sweet corn,[234] nor do I advise their use if you want to be constipation-free.

If you eat these foods, they should be minimized in the diet.

Cooked Foods

"If you eat living food, the same will quicken you, but if you kill your food the dead food will kill you also. For life comes only from life, and from death always comes death." - Attributed to Jesus, *The Essene Gospel of Peace, Book One*.

Nutritional experts have stressed for years that cooked foods are harmful to human health, and that the cooking of foods done at home and in restaurants, and in the food factories that manufacture canned, bottled and jarred foods, reduces the food value of the foods by altering their chemical properties and destroying important food components such as enzymes and nutrients, which also includes vitamins. They also have been telling us that cooked food of almost any kind creates acidity in the body.

It is now known that cooking and the refining and processing of foods are responsible for the development of many of the sicknesses and diseases that plague humankind. As stated previously, Americans eat more cooked food than any people on earth, and spend more money on doctor bills and healthcare than any people on earth, and the two appear to be more than mere coincidence.

The fast food franchises, as well as other eating establishments, grill, fry, bake, and steam-heat their foods, or use dehydrated

---

[234] As explained in the chapter on What Everyone Should Know About Fiber.

foods that have already been refined and processed using these methods.

Robert Morse in his book, *The Detox Miracle Sourcebook*, explains how cooking dramatically decreases the molecular energy of foods, since heat affects the electrons of the food molecules and alters their molecular structure. However, when we eat raw foods, their high electromagnetic energy is transferred to the body and its cells.

Dr. N. W. Walker in many of his books, such as *Colon Health* and *Become Younger*, tells us that foods are demagnetized when they are cooked, and that only living (raw, uncooked) plant foods have the magnetic properties that are needed by the body. He states that the fiber we consume in our diets should be comprised of the fiber or roughage of raw plant foods, and that if this fiber comes from cooked foods, it will be demagnetized, or devitalized, to the extent that it will pass through the system with little or no benefit.

In addition, cooked, starchy foods leave a plaster-like coating on the walls of the large intestine (colon). This coating builds up over time as more of these foods are consumed, which decreases the capacity to absorb vital nutrients and prevents food from being completely digested. More is provided about this in the upcoming section on Starchy Foods.

Cooked food is any food heated above 118° F. It includes almost every kind of food that comes in an airtight sealed package (bag, box, can, jar, bottle, etc.). For comparison purposes, a hot shower is 105° F, typical pasteurization temperature is 160° F, water boils at 212° F, canned foods are heated during the canning process to 240-250° F, and microwave and stove ovens heat foods to 300-500° F.

The Only Cure for Constipation

"Cooked food is dead, and actually unsuitable as nourishment for the digestive processes of all animals, including human beings." - Dr. Ann Wigmore, *Be Your Own Doctor*.

Cooked foods (plant or animal) are foods devoid of life. They require additional energy from the body to be digested and assimilated, energy that could be used for other purposes, such as healing. Cooked foods contain coagulated and unusable proteins and dead enzymes that are toxic to the body.

According to Dr. D. C. Jarvis in his book, *Folk Medicine*, cooking reduces potassium 70% for carrots, onions, potatoes, pumpkin and spinach, 60% for cauliflower, cabbage, peas, asparagus, string beans and Brussel sprouts, and 50% for corn, beets and tomatoes. Potassium is needed for, among other things, the proper functioning of the nervous system.

Cooked foods are tasteless compared to raw foods, which is why cooked foods require condiments, such as salt, pepper and sugar, and combinations of them. Many of the condiments have deleterious effects on the body, including refined sugar and refined salt, as explained in the literature.

Because cooked foods are dead foods and deficient in nutrients, our hunger is not sated when we eat them in small portions, so we overeat. However, overeating is known to be a precursor of many health complications, including obesity and disease.

As stated previously, raw plant foods are foods as-found in nature. They are not cooked or chemically altered, and they do not contain preservatives, artificial colors or flavors. Raw plant foods are living foods with their natural life force properties intact. It is this life force that is imparted to us when we eat raw plant foods.

The Only Cure for Constipation

The dangers of cooked foods discussed so far are sufficient in themselves to justify eliminating all cooked foods from the diet. But cooking of foods has more dangers. If food is browned by heat treatment, such as by broiling, baking or deep frying, dangerous chemicals are created, such as advanced glycation end-products (AGEs), which have been linked to diabetes and heart disease.

Furthermore, nutritional experts assert that cooked food is addictive. Like other addictions, the cooked food addiction gets stronger with continued use. But, like other addictions, it can be overcome by refraining from eating them.

The consensus of modern nutritional experts, including Norman W. Walker, Robert Morse, Arnold Ehret, Theresa Mitchell, Ann Wigmore, Edward Howell, David Wolfe, Herbert M. Shelton, O.L.M. Abramowski, Fred Hirsch, Harvey Diamond, Bernard Jensen, Professor Spira, Kristina Carrillo-Bucaram, Victoria Boutenko, Joe Alexander and Paavo Airola, is that the consumption of cooked foods is detrimental to human health, and that they should not be eaten.

The Importance of Enzymes

Enzymes are life-force factors, biological catalysts that are necessary for life processes. They are substances that make life possible. Enzymes are needed for every chemical reaction that takes place in the body. It is claimed that no mineral, vitamin or hormone can do any work without enzymes. The body's ability to digest and assimilate foods is totally dependent on enzymes.

"I attest that the kitchen stove and its big brothers, the heat treatment machinery in food factories, are responsible for destroying a whole category of food elements, namely the heat-sensitive exogenous food enzymes." - Dr. Edward Howell, *Enzyme Nutrition*.

Whole plant foods are replete with enzymes as provided by nature to facilitate their digestion and assimilation in the body. According to Dr. Edward Howell, raw plant foods have all the enzymes needed for human consumption. The pancreas produces enzymes, but you'll always have exogenous enzymes if you eat raw, uncooked foods.

"To get enzymes from food, one must eat raw food. The heat used in cooking destroys all food enzymes and forces the organism to produce more enzymes, thus enlarging digestive organs, especially the pancreas." - Dr. Edward Howell, *Enzyme Nutrition*.

Nutritional experts believe that eating cooked food requires the body to use up its enzyme reserves for digestion and assimilation. More specifically, the enzymes of the body must perform the job of digesting cooked foods. This depletes the enzyme reserves of the body, making it increasingly difficult as time goes by to properly digest foods. As a result, we become weaker and more fatigued despite the amount of food we consume. In addition, energy that is used by the body to digest cooked foods is diverted away from other badly needed bodily functions such as self-cleansing and healing.

One of the things that interests me in particular about the dangers of eating cooked foods is that Dr. Howell in his book, *Enzyme Nutrition*, states that enzyme activity in the body becomes weaker with age. He also states that based on clinical studies performed on animals and humans, each of us is given a limited supply of enzymes at birth, and that when the supply is depleted, we die, and the faster we use up our enzyme supply the shorter our life will be. This is one of the main reasons why we should avoid all cooked foods. It implies that the more cooked foods we eat, the sooner our life will come to an end.

Again, cooked foods are devoid of enzymes because heat destroys them. Furthermore, cooked foods cause us to look older than we really are. They make wrinkles appear, especially on the face.

Dr. Ann Wigmore, in her book, *Be Your Own Doctor*, states that when food is cooked it permits tumors and cancer growth to build, but when food is eaten raw the cancer and other growths immediately begin to shrink. This indicates that cooked foods are precursors of human disease.

Surprisingly, there is a dearth of information on the Web about the harmful effects of cooked foods on human health.[235] Many of the websites queried for this information actually encourage eating cooked foods as part of a healthy diet. Again, books have the answers to many of the important questions about foods and nutrition.

Whole plant foods may be sliced, diced, run through a food processor, blender, etc., as long as they are not cooked. They can be eaten by themselves or combined with other raw foods if properly combined (see the chapter on Proper Food Combinations).

"Eating raw foods is the number one activity which preserves enzymes and maximizes health." - Gabriel Cousens, *Conscious Eating*.

---

[235] Maybe not so surprisingly if you are familiar with the Internet.

The conclusion is obvious. We should eat as many enzyme-rich foods as possible, which are whole plant foods, and avoid all cooked foods.

David Wolfe in his book, *The Sunfood Diet Success System,* states that it typically takes one month on the diet to reverse one year on a cooked/toxic food diet, to dissolve and eliminate the improper materials that have accumulated in the body. But this schedule, apparently, does not consider the accelerators of periodic fasting and colonics and/or enemas.

The dangers of eating cooked foods may shock or surprise many people because most of us grew up eating cooked foods and have learned to like them. Hopefully, this chapter will serve as a re-thinking starting point about how cooked foods should be viewed.

Substituting living plant foods for cooked foods solves all of the problems described in this chapter.

For more information about how cooked foods are harmful to human health, I refer you to the books listed in the Bibliography by Norman W. Walker, Robert Morse, Arnold Ehret, Theresa Mitchell, Ann Wigmore, Edward Howell, David Wolfe, Herbert M. Shelton, O.L.M. Abramowski, Fred Hirsch, Harvey Diamond, Bernard Jensen, Professor Spira, Kristina Carrillo-Bucaram, Victoria Boutenko, Joe Alexander and Paavo Airola.

Starchy Foods

Two of the most eminent nutritionists of recent times, Professor Arnold Ehret and Dr. Norman W. Walker, made remarkable discoveries of how starchy foods harm the body. They discovered, for example, that patients who habitually eat starchy foods, including pastries and other bread products, rice, and pasta, have clogged up intestines, and. furthermore, that it was the cause of their diseased conditions.

Any starchy food, including macaroni, pizza and potatoes, and cereal products like oats, can be made into paste or plaster. Many of us know this. But what many of us do not know is that the same foods can cause intestinal obstruction to where the passage of wastes becomes completely cut off.

Many people do not know that many starchy and therefore sticky natural foods, even fruits like dates and mangoes, can, especially as ones ages, cause constipation and keep someone from being constipation-free. We need to be aware of these things as we continue to live the constipation-free life.

It was from X-rays and autopsies of people with long histories of poor eating habits, such as eating a lot of cooked and starchy foods, that Dr. Norman W. Walker discovered that the obstructions increase in thickness over time and were caused by the starch plating out on the intestinal lining. A plate-out coated lining of the intestines not only causes constipation, but prevents nutrient exchange to the bloodstream. In time, it builds up to where the passage of waste is so reduced that it is cut off completely, requiring hospitalization and surgery – which often means colostomy. Colostomy is a surgical procedure that involves diverting a piece of the colon to a surgically made opening in the abdominal wall to bypass the clogged up colon.

In other words, constipation caused by starchy foods can be so severe that all waste can be prevented from being expelled from the body, and the only solution according to medical science is surgery. The severe bodily toxicity that such a condition produces causes sickness and disease.

The Only Cure for Constipation

Walker believed that any treatment of disease would be totally ineffective unless the accumulated starchy plaque that has formed in the large intestine over the years has been washed out of the colon by colonic irrigations. This conclusion is based on his healing of chronically ill patients by having them undergo a series of colonics. It was the cleansing action of the colonics that caused the plaque to be released from the walls of the colon, and when that occurred the health of his patients was restored. This is exactly what Arnold Ehret and others have stressed in their books.

For years I ate whatever foods were sold and whatever I wanted in the days of innocence when I didn't know any better. But I know better now because my quest for living constipation-free has led me to good books about what really causes it and what foods to avoid to be constipation- and disease-free. In fact, as discussed in this book, the two go hand in hand, for when you cure constipation you effectively eliminate one of the main causes of disease. I can feel what starchy foods do to me every time I eat them, so I no longer eat them.

The clogging up of the intestines caused by starchy foods causes intestinal bacteria to multiply inordinately, which releases poisons into the blood stream. The state of constipation is the primary cause of illness and disease in the human body also according to Professor Arnold Ehret, Dr. Ann Wigmore, Fred Hirsch, Karyn Calabrese, Professor Spira, and other noted nutritionists.

Many of the contributors to our understanding of the causes of human diseases were famous nutritionists, including Professor Arnold Ehret, who was, as mentioned previously, popular in Germany in the early 1900s, and later in America.

Ehret was probably the first scientist to recognize that mucus-forming foods cause waste obstruction in the body, and that the obstruction causes disease. As stated previously, in his book, *The Cause and Cure of Human Illness*, he states that there are two main reasons for human disease: 1) constipation caused by mucus-producing foods, and 2) overeating, i.e., eating more than is necessary, more than the system can handle, more than it actually needs.

As stated previously, in his landmark book, *The Mucusless Diet Healing System*, first published in 1922, Ehret believed that optimum health is achieved by eating a starch-free diet consisting of fresh raw fruits, leafy greens and non-starchy vegetables (mucusless foods) which he claimed was the optimal diet for human health. These are the natural foods of man (Genesis' "fruits and herbs"). The book is considered by many nutritional experts to be the definitive work on the prevention and curing of human disease through diet and fasting.

Some of the dangers of eating starchy foods have been discussed in the chapter on the Causes of Disease. As mentioned in that chapter, Ehret healed himself of Bright's disease (a kidney disease), and cured many hopeless cases of chronic diseases by putting his patients on his mucusless diet and fasting regimen. Many of the patients were very serious cases with terminal diseases, and lay on their deathbeds. Many had gone through other therapies and followed the advice given, including strict diets, but without success. He also cured those who suffered from degenerative diseases, both acute and chronic. After following his mucusless diet for only a short time, all of his patients regained their health.

Starchy foods include wheat, oats, corn, rice, white and red potatoes, but also beans of all kinds and peas. They also include food products made from these foods, such as bread, pasta, cereals, pastries, corn starch, etc. (Note that carrots and beets are non-starchy foods, as discussed in the chapter on Proper Food Combinations.)

Many websites claim that eating fiber foods, such as grains, is important for general health and elimination of constipation. While that is true, an *overconsumption of fiber foods* can cause GI problems, including constipation and hemorrhoids, as explained in the chapter on What Everyone Should Know About Fiber.

Grains are also high in starch, and starch is known for causing constipation that leads to disease.[236] [237] For example, online sources claim that cornmeal is 74% starch, wholewheat bread is 58%, refined grains such as white bread and bread flour 40-44%, and potatoes 18% starch.[238] These foods are staples in many American households.

Don't wait until you are constipated to do something about it. Start now to severely cut back on the foods that are proven to cause constipation.

Many people are not aware of the dangers of starchy foods, as they are not aware of the dangers of cooked foods. It is amazing that, at the time of this writing, I could not find any websites that discussed the harmful effects that starches have on the large intestine (colon), or that attribute starchy foods to causing disease. It seems that starchy foods are so much a part of our culture that no one wants to hear the truth about them.

"If you consumed a lifetime supply of dairy, meat and other

---

[236] Arnold Ehret, <u>The Mucusless Diet Healing System</u>.
[237] Norman W. Walker, <u>Colon Health</u>.
[238] https://www.healthline.com/nutrition/high-starch-foods#.

mucus-producing foods, you may have built up many layers of glue-like toxins on your colon walls. Although some waste can pass through your intestines daily, leading you to believe that your body is adequately digesting the food you eat, the lining of your intestines will continue to toughen and narrow." - Karyn Calabrese, *Soak Your Nuts*.

"No system of healing can be permanently effective until the eliminative organs have been thoroughly cleansed of accumulated waste matter and at the same time all grain and starchy foods have been eliminated from one's diet." - Norman W. Walker, *Become Younger*.

The clogging up process resulting from the consumption of starchy foods can be easily proven on a whole plant food diet by simply eating, for a short time, white flour products, such as pizza or while flour bread. The result is constipation and difficult bowel movements, whereas avoiding these foods results in the return to regular and smooth defecations.

Let me ask you a simple question. Are you sure you want to eat that next slice of bread or bowl of rice?

Oils

Oils, like fats, require long digestion times. Despite the hype about oils being good for heath, they are bad for heath because they cause constipation. When constipation-free, try eating just one corn chip or potato chip and you will see the dire results.

Painkillers

Painkillers, such as NSAIDs (Nonsteroidal Anti-inflammatory Drugs) and opioids, are known to worsen chronic constipation.

NSAIDs work by blocking enzymes called cyclooxygenase (or COX), which are prostaglandins, or fatty acids or their derivatives known as lipids, that are produced at sites of tissue damage or infection that control pain and inflammation.[239] The gastrointestinal (GI) side effects of NSAIDs include bleeding, weakening of the intestinal lining, ulceration of the large intestine and leaky gut syndrome or intestinal permeability. NSAIDs also increase the risk of stomach ulcers and ulcers of the duodenum, which is the first part of the small intestine.[240] In addition, they weaken the immune system by inhibiting antibody production in cells,[241] meaning that NSAIDs increase the risk of getting infections.

In addition, irritation of the GI tract caused by NASIDs can lead to colitis or the worsening of a preexisting colonic disease.[242]

A 2020 Web article entitled, "NSAIDs Cause Osteoarthritis," by Fred D. Arnold, NMD,[243] states that numerous scientific studies have shown that patients who use NSAIDs to treat osteoarthritis (OA) have increased cartilage breakdown that leads to the need for joint replacements. It also states that it is the massive use of NSAIDs in patients with OA during the past forty years that has led to the rapid rise in the need for hip and knee replacements, as revealed in the HCUP statistical brief that was cited in the last chapter. In addition, it states that over 100,000 people are hospitalized for GI bleeding, and 16,500 die from NSAID toxicity each year.

---

[239] https://www.betterhealth.vic.gov.au/health/conditionsandtreatme.
[240] Elizabeth Lipski, Ph.D., CCN, Digestive Wellness.
[241] https://www.ncbi.nlm.nih.gov/pmc/articles/PMC2693360/.
[242] https://pubmed.ncbi.nlm.nih.gov/8739836/#:~:text=Non-steroidal%20anti-inflammatory.
[243] http://www.prolotherapyphoenix.com › Article-NSAID.

Chapter 15 Abiding by Nature's Laws

Natural laws govern our world. They include the laws of physics that encompass the mysterious forces of electromagnetism, gravity and the nuclear forces, and also the laws of biological processes, including life itself. Natural laws are always in effect, and they apply to everyone in every generation.

All creatures seem to be perfectly attuned and adjusted to these laws, except for man. We are constantly challenging or testing Nature in one way or another. Our free will, which other creatures do not have, and which sets us apart from the other creatures perhaps more than anything else, enables us to question the validity of natural laws. But Nature has a way of punishing and even eliminating those who break her laws.

In the province of Nature, things happen to us as a consequence of the way that we choose to live, the choices that we make in life, including our food choices and eating habits. For example, if I combine my foods improperly, I can expect a stomachache or headache. If I eat the Standard American Diet, I can expect to be the recipient of a large number of food-related health disorders that are linked to meat and dairy products and to devitalized, refined and processed foods.

The law of cause and effect is one of Nature's laws. It happens to be the foundation of the scientific method, which is the basis for all the discoveries and inventions made in the sciences, including chemistry, physics, geology, biology and the medical sciences. The law of cause and effect is observed in many clinical trials and studies conducted on human health and nutrition each year that show a direct link between the diseases of humankind and diet. Some of these trials and studies are documented in articles of the scientific and medical professions, many of which are available online, and some are cited in this book as well as the books that are listed in the Bibliography.

If you don't want the effects, do something about the causes.

"The present ignorance of the laws underlying normal health is now, in this century, the greatest of all the past centuries, and is evidenced by the deterioration of the so-called civilized people health-wise." - Arnold Ehret, *Physical Fitness Through a Superior Diet, Fasting, and Dietetics*.

As discussed in the chapter on the Causes of Disease, many medical researchers and nutritionists claim that the cause of many human diseases are the foods that are commonly consumed, rather than normal processes of aging, such as natural "wear and tear" on the body. It is my belief that this claim will be proven to everyone's satisfaction in the years to come, impacting many popular beliefs regarding age-related health issues. An example is the degenerative disease of arthritis. Many nutritionists, including Dr. Ann Wigmore, believe that arthritis is caused by harmful dietary practices.[244]

Fasting (simply eating less) is one of Nature's powerful ways of cleansing the body of the harmful effects of improper diet and too much eating. When animals get sick, they instinctively abstain from food. But man seems to have lost this instinct, if he ever had it.

It is our duty to understand Nature's laws if we wish to live a healthy life, one that is free of health disorders, including diseases like constipation. The appreciation of the power of a natural law at

---

[244] For additional information, see S. H. Shepherd, The Cure for Arthritis.

work in us is one of the most profound things that we can ever experience.

Eating foods with their enzymes intact, undestroyed by heat (whole plant foods), avoiding the dangers of cooked and starchy foods, learning proper food combinations, and curing health issues through a combination of proper diet and fasting are only a few examples of dietary practices that adhere to the laws of Nature.

Another law of nature is the need for adequate rest. As mentioned previously, in our fast-paced society with its unrelenting demands on our time and money, our minds cry out for adequate rest. We are told that eight hours of sleep per night are required for health, but many of us get less than five. Is this abiding by Nature's laws?

Also as stated previously, the body always lets us know how we are treating it. Understanding and heeding the warning signals the body provides helps us to maintain ourselves in concert with the laws of nature. As mentioned previously, the body can take a lot of abuse before it starts to show the ill effects of deterioration. But when that occurs, a person could be, health-wise speaking, at the point of no return. By staying proactive in this regard, we can avoid many of the health disorders, including diseases, that stalk our society.

Chapter 16 Obesity

We have an obesity epidemic in this country. It is due to several factors, not all of which will be discussed here, but the main factors will be covered. One of the main causes for the epidemic is the consumption of saturated fats found in meat and dairy products, and many refined and processed foods, including, but not limited to, snack foods. Because these foods are deficient in nutrients and enzymes, our body's need for nutrients, and our hunger, is not satisfied when we eat them, so we overeat, which compounds the problem.

Technically speaking, the term "obesity" is used to describe people who have a body mass index (BMI) greater than 30.[245] BMI is a measure of body fat based on height and weight and is applicable to adult men and women. Tables of BMI online allow anyone to determine their BMI.[246]

Overeating is so common in the US that it is considered normal, even though it is a precursor of many health disorders. An old saying is that you will find many people who are old, and many people who are overweight or obese, but you will not find many who are old and overweight or obese. It is because being overweight or obese shortens life span.

It is well known that the more overweight or obese a person is, the more likely he or she will develop a disease – any disease – including constipation, but also high blood pressure. When overweight or obese, the heart must work harder than normal to pump the blood through the arteries and blood vessels to the

---

[245] https://www.nhlbi.nih.gov/health/educational/lose_wt/BMI/bmicalc.
[246] Ibid.

organs and tissues of the body, which increases blood pressure. Additionally, high blood pressure caused by an overweight or obese condition damages the tiny blood vessels in the kidneys.[247]

Overeating is so widespread that I sought additional reasons that might explain the epidemic. One of the reasons appears to be the pride or hubris that is associated with having a plentiful supply of foods. We don't face starvation in this country, just the choice between a Whopper and a Big Mac. We have more food than anyone needs or can possibly use, and in such an unrivaled variety of products. It is a supply that others in the world do not have. So, why pass up the opportunity to indulge, while you still can? Such thinking leads to ill health.

It is only logical that there is a direct relationship between obesity and constipation, for each depends in large part, if not totally, on the foods we eat.

As stated previously, the quantity of food consumed during meals also matters for health. Nutritionists, such as Dr. Robert Morse, Ann Wigmore, Edward Howell and Herbert M. Shelton, believe that digestive juices are secreted not in proportion to the amount of food eaten, but in proportion to the amount of food that is required by the system. (This may change your opinion about overeating.)

As an obese person, or any other person, continues to overeat, their system becomes more and more clogged up, choked with internal undigested waste material. The resulting putrefaction causes bodily acidity and produces toxins that pollute the blood, a condition known as bodily toxicity.

---

[247] https://www.healthgrades.com › weight-control-and-obesity.

The Only Cure for Constipation

Gluttony can cause obesity. The dictionary defines gluttony as habitual greed or excess in eating. Instead of overeating because the body senses a lack of nutrients in the foods, the glutton desires more food just to feel full, or for no particular reason at all. From a science of nutrition point of view, gluttony may be defined as habitually eating in excess of the body's supply of gastric juices. The Bible frowns on gluttony, treating it like drunkenness.

"Our greatest desire in life is retaining "youth" – with its grace, beauty, vivacity, and charm! But through wrong eating, gluttony, and faulty elimination, we are old at 40!" - Professor Arnold Ehret, *Thus Speaketh the Stomach and the Tragedy of Nutrition*.

An overweight or obese condition can be corrected through exercise, which burns up calories that otherwise would turn into fat. It can also be corrected by dietary change. The choices are available to anyone. However, recognizing the many health hazards associated with being overweight is not all that it takes for many people to seriously want to change the way they eat and also quite possibly the way they live. One must first come to grips with why they are compulsive eaters. Looking inside ourselves for the answers is perhaps the most difficult thing of all to do, especially for those who are obese.

The reasons for overindulging are many and must first be faced and dealt with, for it is well known that many obese people never change their ways of eating just by adopting a diet or exercising more often.

Nevertheless, since exercise boosts the metabolism and enhances health in so ways other than the correction of an overweight condition, it must be considered in any alternative heath strategy. According to the CDC, losing as little as 5 to 10 percent of body weight can have substantial health benefits,[248] and, by following a calorie deficit diet or a program of intermittent fasting, one can substantially reduce their body fat and thereby lower their BMI level.[249]

---

[248] https://www.everydayhealth.com/diet-nutrition/bmi/how-you-reduce-your-bmi-science-backed.
[249] https://www.northhoustonclinic.com/how-to-lower-bmi-5-medically-proven-ways-to-lose-weight/#:~:text=By%20following%2.

Chapter 17 Colonics and Enemas

"Death begins in the colon." - Elie Metchnikoff.

Nutritional experts contend that many of the problems we are now facing, including age-related health disorders, are due to the condition of our colons. But they go further and tell us that many, if not most, diseases of humankind *originate* in the colon. This incredible assertion is explained in the books by Arnold Ehret, Dr. Ann Wigmore and Dr. N. W. Walker that are listed in the Bibliography, and is supported by other nutritional experts.

"Your constitutional encumbrances throughout the entire system are the source of every disease; the greatest and most harmful source of lowered vitality, imperfect health, lack of strength and endurance and any and all imperfect conditions. All have their source in the colon, never perfectly emptied since your birth." - Arnold Ehret, *The Mucusless Diet Healing System*.

Hippocrates said, "All disease begins in the gut."

What if we acted on this information? If there is a direct link between the diseases of humankind and the condition of the colon, shouldn't we do whatever is possible to eliminate toxic waste buildup and the plate-out of starchy plaque in the colon? Of course we should, and each of us can.

Colonics and enemas help remove the plaque-like deposits in our colons and release and move toxins out of our systems. In this way, they accelerate the self-cleansing and healing process of the body. Nutritional experts Arnold Ehret, Dr. Norman Walker and others consider colonics and enemas either absolutely necessary or highly advantageous for healing chronic diseases.

The Only Cure for Constipation

If you have never had a colonic or enema, you are not alone. Most people have never had them, and many have never even heard of them. However, as we journey to optimum health we become more and more our own doctors. The transition to a whole plant food diet is the time to learn about these procedures and how to perform them.

Colonics (also known as colon irrigations or colon hydrotherapy), are procedures performed in the privacy of a personal suite at a local colonic establishment. They help clean out the toxins and wastes accumulated in the colon.

Colonic establishments are located in most cities. The average cost for a colonic irrigation (or hydrotherapy) ranges $60-$100 and you can purchase multiple sessions to save money. I have done the colon hydrotherapy several times. The machine is self-operated and easy to use. You can control it at your own pace for as long as you want. For me, that was about 30 minutes. I decided on the colonics after I read the books by Dr. N.W. Walker, and particularly his book, *Become Younger*.

A less expensive way to assist the detoxification process is to perform enemas at home. Enema kits are available at most retail stores (Wal-Mart, drug stores, etc.). Each kit has a number of small plastic bottles that contain a saline solution. The procedure is to lie down, turn on one side and insert the tip of the bottle and squeeze the bottle. I discovered that best results are obtained by replacing half of the saline solution with freshly-squeezed lemon juice, and using 2 bottles at a time instead of one.

Other types of enema kits are available, such as the travel-bag variety which consists of a long plastic tube and a plastic bag that hangs from a door knob.

The Only Cure for Constipation

Doing enemas is a good, positive change to make in your life. It is a learning experience that many would much rather avoid, but again, you are becoming more and more your own doctor as you continue on the health journey.

If you have less than three bowel movements a day then you should be doing colonics and/or enemas on a more frequent basis than once a month. Otherwise, once a month is recommended.

Colonics and enemas are not coffee table topics for discussion. They are real-world procedures that need to be understood if anyone is serious about achieving optimum health.

For a more thorough discussion of the need for colonics and enemas, see the books by Arnold Ehret and N.W. Walker in the Bibliography.

"My experience during the past ten years has proven, by the rapid recovery of all diseases after the colon was cleansed, that in the colon itself lies the basic cause of almost all human ailments." - Arnold Ehret, *The Definite Cure of Chronic Constipation*.

Remember, if it were possible to attain optimum health and longevity without knowledge or effort or discernment whatsoever on the part of the individual, then everyone would be wonderfully healthy. If optimum health could be sold as a magic pill or silver bullet, then anyone could become healthy without the slightest effort. But all things are given to us at the expenditure of effort.

Remember, also, as discussed in the chapter on the Causes of Disease, that many nutritionists contend that many, if not most, of the diseases of humankind originate in the colon.

The Only Cure for Constipation

"The "basement" of the human "temple" is the reservoir from which every symptom of disease and weakness is supplied in all its manifestations." - Arnold Ehret, *The Mucusless Diet Healing System*.

If people would incorporate the information contained in this chapter in their lives, they would be doing their health a great service, and perhaps more than they may realize.

Chapter 18 What Everyone Should Know About Fiber

This chapter discusses what dietary fiber does for constipation, and for health in general. Dietary fiber, sometimes called roughage, comes only from plants.[250] [251] All fruits, vegetables, nuts and seeds have fiber. Foods that do not have fiber are meat products, including beef, pork, poultry and fish, eggs, milk, yogurt, all types of cheese and all other dairy products. In other words, animal-based foods are devoid of fiber.

Fiber is basically either soluble and insoluble. Most plant foods contain both types. Insoluble fiber passes through the system undigested; most people are referring to insoluble fiber when it is discussed in the literature.

Soluble fiber dissolves in water and is digestible, meaning, among other things, that it is good for gut microbiota. Soluble fiber has other benefits too; it helps lower blood cholesterol and balance blood sugar, whereas insoluble fiber does not do these things.

Insoluble fiber, such as the cellulose in plants, adds bulk to stools which helps move wastes along. Soluble fiber induces intestinal contractions (peristalsis) which also helps move wastes along. Therefore, both types assist in eliminating constipation, and in doing so decrease a person's risk of getting other intestinal

---

[250] https://extension.usu.edu/archive/is-all-dietary-fiber-the-same#:~:text=Dietary%20fiber%20is%20found%20only,as%20those%20that%20are%20raw.

[251] https://www.mayoclinic.org/healthy-lifestyle/nutrition-and-healthy-eating/in-depth/fiber/art-20043983#:~:text=Dietary%20fiber%2C%20also%20known%20as,t%20digested%20by%20your%20body.

disorders, including colon cancer, diarrhea, hemorrhoids and Irritable Bowel Syndrome. [252] [253] [254] [255] [256] [257] [258] [259]

As stated in a 2017 National Center for Biotechnology Information (NBCI) report:

"Insoluble dietary fiber increases fecal mass and accelerates colonic transit via mechanical stimulation/irritation of the colonic mucosa with increasing secretion and peristalsis. Soluble dietary fiber is fermented by bacteria in the large intestine, which increases the stool bulk by increasing the biomass by fermentation byproducts such as gas and short-chain fatty acids."[260]

According to a 2019 NBCI Report:

"Epidemiological studies have shown that diets which are high in fat, sugar, and salt, and low in dietary fiber can predispose the consumer to the many chronic diseases of our time, such as diabetes, obesity, cardiovascular disease, certain cancers and more."[261]

Human dietary guidelines for years have stressed the need to

---

[252] https://www.livestrong.com/article/464063-what-foods-contain-cellulose/.
[253] https://www.katefarms.com/articles/featured-articles/soluble-fiber/.
[254] https://www.healthline.com/nutrition/benefits-of-cabbage#:~:text.
[255] https://healthyeating.sfgate.com/amount-fiber-baked-potato-skin-6736.html.
[256] https://www.gicare.com/gi-health-resources/prebiotics/.
[257] https://www.bodybuildingindia.com/blogs/blog/10-benefits-of-sweet-corn
[258] https://www.hsph.harvard.edu/nutritionsource/carbohydrates/fiber/.
[259] https://www.seacoastonline.com/story/lifestyle/health-fitness/2020/09/10/put-away-peeler-skins-add-nutritional-value/113763314/.
[260] https://www.ncbi.nlm.nih.gov/pmc/articles/PMC5548066/.
[261] https://www.ncbi.nlm.nih.gov/pmc/articles/PMC6537190/.

make fruits and vegetables a substantial part of one's diet. Fruits and vegetables have always been promoted for their vitamins, especially vitamins C and A, and minerals, but they are more recently being promoted for their dietary fiber and phytochemicals (antioxidants).

Foods high in insoluble fiber include brown rice, whole wheat, rye and barley breads, multigrain breads, celery, cabbage, cauliflower, corn, broccoli, potatoes, carrots, zucchini, mushrooms, and leafy greens such as spinach and lettuce. Most websites agree that whole wheat bread has about 80% insoluble fiber, wheat bran 100% insoluble fiber, split peas 100%, potatoes 70%, broccoli 87%, kidney beans and pinto beans 80%, corn (like kernel corn), 90%, brown rice, grits and oatmeal 75%, and avocados 82% insoluble fiber. [262] [263]

Some sources say fruits such as apples and pears, mangoes, figs, bananas and raisins are high in insoluble fiber, but others say they are high in soluble fiber. I believe that without the skins they are mostly soluble fiber.

Foods high in soluble fiber besides those identified above include beans, nuts and seeds, garlic, oatmeal and oat bran, berries and the citrus fruits, including oranges, grapefruit and lemons (without the skins, of course).[264] [265] [266] [267]

---

[262] https://healthyeating.sfgate.com/amount-fiber-baked-potato-skin-6736.html.
[263] https://healthyeating.sfgate.com/increase-insoluble-fiber-intake-5887.html.
[264] https://www.wellandgood.com/foods-high-in-soluble-fiber/.
[265] https://www.medicalnewstoday.com/articles/319176#:~:text.
[266] https://www.realsimple.com/health/nutrition-diet/healthy-eating/soluble-fiber-vs-insoluble-fiber#:.
[267] https://www.mayoclinic.org/healthy-lifestyle/nutrition-and-healthy-eating/in-depth/fiber/art-20043983.

What Type of Fiber is Best for Health?

According to what I have read, no one has come out and claimed definitely that either type of fiber is the best for health or for remedying GI problems. Many nutritional sources treat them as being equally beneficial. [268] [269] [270]

The FDA ruled In 2016 that the fiber listed on Nutrition and Supplement Facts labels should mean *insoluble* fiber, which, for all intents and purposes, equates "fiber" or "dietary fiber" with insoluble fiber.[271] [272] This needs to be taken into account when finding the soluble and insoluble fiber in foods.

The USDA recommends that everyone young and old consume three times more insoluble fiber than soluble fiber.[273] [274] It should be remembered that nutritional guidelines are designed for the majority of people, and, while well intended, they may not be what is best for *all* people. Since each person is a unique creation, having slightly different needs, and likes and dislikes, for foods, etc., one type of fiber may be better than another for health depending on the individual.

I have found that it's best to eat a *combination* of soluble and insoluble fibers, which is, in any case, what you get when you eat an almost all fruit and vegetable diet.

---

[268] Ibid.
[269] https://www.medicalnewstoday.com/articles/does-soluble-fat-bind-cholesterol#binding-to-cholesterol.
[270] https://healthyeating.sfgate.com/zero-fiber-food-7968.html.
[271] https://www.fda.gov/food/food-labeling-nutrition/questions-and-answers-dietary-fiber.
[272] https://www.verywellfit.com/learn-about-dietary-fiber-2506531.
[273] https://www.katefarms.com/articles/featured-articles/soluble-fiber/.
[274] Elizabeth Lipski, Ph.D., CCN, Digestive Wellness.

The Only Cure for Constipation

For example, corn, cauliflower and mushrooms have mostly insoluble fiber. Cabbage, cucumbers, onions and prunes have about an equal amount of soluble and insoluble fiber. Peeled apples and bananas have mostly soluble fiber. [275] [276] [277]

If you've been constipated for years from eating foods of the traditional or standard American diet but have not undergone detoxification to reduce your accumulated waste and bodily toxins, then your gut ecosystem probably requires work, indicating that before improvement can be seen in your condition, the diversity of your gut microbiota must be boosted. In that case, you should eat more soluble fiber, at least at first. Also, if you are sensitive to digesting grains, then you should include more soluble fiber foods in your diet since grains are typically high in insoluble fiber.[278]

It is also important to know the starch content of foods because of its direct connection with constipation. In fact, the starch content alone may override any benefit obtained from eating fiber foods.[279]

Additionally, too much insoluble fiber in the diet can induce or exacerbate a constipated condition, particularly in the elderly.

"Paradoxically, high fiber foods can constipate you." - Dr. Judy Nee, M.D., Harvard Medical School and Beth Israel Deaconess Medical Center.[280]

---

[275] https://www.healthline.com/nutrition/benefits-of-cabbage#:~:text.
[276] https://healthyeating.sfgate.com/carbs-fiber-raw-onion-6288.html.
[277] https://www.realsimple.com/health/nutrition-diet/healthy-eating/soluble-fiber-vs-insoluble-fiber#:
[278] https://www.realsimple.com/health/nutrition-diet/healthy-eating/soluble-fiber-vs-insoluble-fiber#:
[279] The dangers of eating starchy foods are discussed in Chapter 14.
[280] https://www.consumerreports.org/medical-conditions/how-to-relieve-constipation/.

Another fact to consider about the fiber in foods is what we do to foods. Peeling fruits and vegetables will reduce their fiber, so to get more fiber eat the skins, such as on apples. As for cooking, some sources say it reduces the fiber in foods; for example. it is said that uncooked broccoli has about 87% insoluble fiber (as indicated previously), but it reduces to 60% when cooked because cellulose, one of the main types of insoluble fiber found in vegetables, is degraded by heat.[281] [282] Other sources claim that cooking concentrates the fiber in foods.[283] Still other sources claim that neither is so, as indicated in the following quotation.

"Cooking does not change the amount of fiber in foods; cooked and puréed vegetables contain the same amount of fiber as raw vegetables."[284]

In many cases, we must prove, through trial and error, what is best for us rather than relying on what others say who are supposedly in the know.

<u>The Benefits of Sweet Corn</u>

One of the most versatile of all foods is corn, which contains mostly insoluble fiber, as does popcorn. Classified by botanists as a fruit, corn is commonly considered a vegetable or a grain.[285] It is more affordable than most other vegetables, yet higher in nutrients, including protein. Additionally, it is good for gluten-intolerant people because it is gluten free.[286]

---

[281] Ibid.
[282] https://healthyeating.sfgate.com/increase-insoluble-fiber-intake-5887.html.
[283] https://www.ncbi.nlm.nih.gov/pmc/articles/PMC6537190/.
[284] Ibid.
[285] https://marinmg.ucanr.edu/files/141899.pdf.
[286] https://www.ehow.com/info_8624619_differences-between-maize-corn.html.

The Only Cure for Constipation

"Today, corn is inescapable, consumed with intent and by accident in equal measure." - Reuters.

At the time of this writing, most whole sweet corn and all popcorn are not genetically modified organisms (GMO).[287] However, corn of the GMO variety is widely used in refined and processed foods as either "sugar" or high-fructose corn syrup (HFCS).[288] [289]

The health hazards of eating GMO foods such as GMO corn, has been hotly debated, and yet there are no requirements for labeling whether a food item is or is not genetically engineered. The private sector tries to do this job but upwards of 75% of the refined and processed foods on supermarket shelves contain unlabeled GMO products. For more information, including a current list of foods that are GMO, see the footnoted reference. [290]

Sweet corn is easily expelled which, as discussed previously, makes for less constipation, better sleeps and better overall health. As can easily be seen in the toilet, corn in kernel form is mostly expelled as waste, so only a small percentage of the kernels are digested, most going right through the system and making for softer stools because of their fiber. However, cornmeal, cornbread and other corn products, which are high in both fiber and starch, worsen constipation.

Being human means having problems to solve, but the better

---

[287] https://www.ewg.org/news-insights/news/most-corn-cob-isnt-gmo#:~:text=Most%20sweet%20corn%20has%20not,particularly%20over%20the%20long%20term.

[288] https://www.ewg.org/news-insights/news/most-corn-cob-isnt-gmo#:~:text=Most%20sweet%20corn%20has%20not,particularly%20over%20the%20long%20term.

[289] https://www.huffpost.com/entry/corn-health-myths-nutrition_n_5591977.

[290] Stan Shepherd, Raw Veganism.

informed we are about the problems, the better we can deal with them.

Whole sweet corn is more than 90% insoluble fiber.[291] Its starch content, some websites claim, is 18%.[292] But, again, it depends on what source is used for the reference. For example, several online sources say that the starch content of corn is 28–80% of its dry weight.[293] Others say it is 61%.[294]

However, if we do our own calculations by using the starch equation given in the chapter on Proper Food Combinations, and use gram weights of the food components obtained from their Nutrition Facts Labels, we arrive at a much lower value for the starch in sweet corn, which I believe is the correct value, as seen below.

Example 1:

For a serving of 1/2 cup of sweet corn (given as 76.5g), net carbs are 14.3g, sugar 4.7g and fiber 2g.[295]

Starch = Carbs – (Sugars + Fiber)

So starch = 14.3g - (4.7g + 2g) = 6.7 divided by 1/2 cup (= 76.5g) = 7.6g/76.5g = 10%, half of what most sources claim, and they no doubt get their information from other sources, which compounds the uncertainly.

---

[291] https://healthyeating.sfgate.com/increase-insoluble-fiber-intake-5887.html.
[292] https://www.healthline.com/nutrition/high-starch-foods.
[293] https://www.healthline.com/nutrition/foods/corn#nutrients.
[294] According to https://www.sciencedirect.com/science/article/pii, corn kernels have 61%–78% starch on a dry basis.
[295] https://www.carbmanager.com/food-detail/cc:fab0b76bc35044c280 785da5b3f2ad96/corn-yellow-and-white-cooked-from-fresh-whole-kernel.

The Only Cure for Constipation

<u>Example 2</u>:

For a serving of 3.5 oz (100g) sweet corn, carbs are 21g, sugar 4.5g and fiber 2.4g.[296]

Starch = Carbs – (Sugars + Fiber) = 21g - (4.5g + 2.4g) = 6.9, say 7g, divided by 3.5 oz (100g) = 7g/100g = <u>7%</u>.

The takeaway is that you can do your own analysis of the starch content of foods and do not have to rely on what others say, and also that the starch content of sweet corn, such as frozen kernel corn, is no more than 10%, despite what online sources say.

Both sweet kernel corn and popcorn act as "intestinal brooms" that assist in sweeping out long-deposited starchy plaque from the lining of the intestines.[297] Obviously, we should eat these foods, as long as *no* butter or oils are used on them. Ergo, air pop.

Wholewheat bread and oats have about 58% starch. The starch content of other breads is 40-44%, and cooked pasta is 26% starch.[298] As explained in Chapter 14, the starch begins its deadly plate-out deposit work in the body as soon as it reaches the intestines, which makes it difficult for foods to be fully digested and clogs up the system. Starchy foods are a main contributor to constipation and hinder food transit time, which increases the chances of getting other GI problems, like hemorrhoids. Which are worse for constipation, fats/oils or starchy foods like breads? Initially, fats/oils because of their long digestion times, but both are in the long run harm the body.

---

[296] https://www.healthline.com/nutrition/foods/corn#nutrients.
[297] https://www.cookinglight.com/eating-smart/nutrition-101/fiber-fundamentals.
[298] https://www.healthline.com/nutrition/high-starch-foods.

Chapter 19 The Blood

"The life of the flesh is in the blood." - Lev. 17:11.

This chapter describes the effects that foods have on blood health and shows how to interpret your own blood condition.

Blood is life. As the poets claim, it is the song of the lark, the blush on the cheek, the spring of the lamb. It is the sacred wine in the silver chalice. Down through the ages, blood has been the price men paid for freedom, and so it is today. Blood is our most preciously guarded possession.

Nutritionists tell us that the quality of the blood starts changing within a few hours after eating a meal. Blood cells, like other cells of the body, are continually being replaced. Old cells are being replaced by new cells. The new cells are constructed from the raw materials that foods and drinks provide. The quality of the blood depends a great deal on the quality of the foods that are eaten. When we eat cooked foods, including refined and processed foods, blood cells are constructed of inferior-quality building materials, materials that are devoid of the life force properties that whole plant foods possess.

"Dead atoms and dead molecules cannot rejuvenate or re-generate the cells of the body. Such food results in cell starvation and this in turn causes sickness and disease." - Norman W. Walker, *Water Can Undermine Your Health*.

As discussed in the chapter on the Causes of Disease, acidity is a blood condition mainly brought on by eating too many acid-producing foods. When we eat foods typical of a cooked meat and/or pasteurized milk diet, which are acidic foods, the blood becomes thick and heavy which causes clogging in the tissues and is known to adversely affect the arteries and lymphatic system, and cause poor circulation and elevated blood pressure. When we eat whole plant foods, such as raw fruits, vegetables and leafy greens, the blood's condition becomes normal, which is alkaline, and is not thickened which results in improved circulation and reduced blood pressure.

Several independent researchers have shown that high dietary acid may be linked to kidney disease.[299]

"Animal foods cannot build good blood; in fact, do not build human blood at all, because of the biological fact that man is by nature a fruit eater. Look at the juice of a ripe blackberry, black cherry or black grapes. Doesn't it almost resemble your blood? Can any reasonable man prove that half-decayed "muscle tissue" builds better blood?" - Arnold Ehret, *Mucusless Diet Healing System*.

Almost all raw plant foods are alkaline, or become alkaline in the body. Fruits of the Citrus genus (oranges, grapefruit, etc.) are alkalizing in the body despite their initial acidity. If we ate nothing but raw fruits, leafy greens and vegetables, our blood chemistry would be alkaline most of the time. The times when it would not be so would be in times of stress, or when we are exposed to environmental toxins, or are taking alcohol, caffeine or medication. Grains, most legumes, and most commonly eaten nuts are acid-forming (and mucus-forming) foods to some extent.

The chlorophyll in leafy green vegetables cleanses and alkalizes the blood. The body converts chlorophyll into heme, an iron compound that is part of hemoglobin, to produce red blood cells.

---

[299] https://www.jhsph.edu/news/news-releases/2016/diet%20-designed-to-lower-blood-pressure-also-reduces-risk%20of-kidney-disease.html.

The Only Cure for Constipation

Unfortunately, many Americans do not eat greens except in small amounts, such as lettuce in fast food sandwiches, which is one of the reasons why many people in this country are lacking in vitamins, antioxidants, and the therapeutic properties that plant foods have. Greens include spinach, kale, chard, lettuces, cabbages, collard greens and mustard greens. The importance of eating greens for health is discussed throughout this book.

Homeostasis, the tendency of the body to maintain itself in stable chemical equilibrium, is critical for proper functioning of the human body. Health is said to be a balancing act, with the body trying to balance or stabilize itself to a normal or alkaline blood condition. Obviously, the effectiveness at doing this is encumbered or enhanced by the foods that are eaten, and how they are eaten.

An acidic blood condition is typically caused by a meat and dairy diet. If the diet is continued, the blood condition worsens to where the body's attempts at homeostasis are not sufficient in neutralizing the acidic condition. The acids the body cannot neutralize and expel as waste get stored in the tissues and joints of the body which can lead to diseases. Meat and grain products are the most acid-forming foods, whereas fruits and vegetables are the most acid-binding foods.[300]

Two examples of the effects of a poor blood condition are anemia, a condition of not having enough healthy red blood cells, and deep-vein thrombosis, which is blood clotting. Healthy blood does not produce these disorders. According to Dr. Michael Greger's book, *How Not to Die*, plant-based diets have been shown to reduce the risk of blood cancers by 50%.

---

[300] Berg's Tables, which provide a listing of what foods are acid-forming and acid-binding, are given in Appendix I.

The Only Cure for Constipation

pH Balance

Nature's way is for the human body to maintain its blood in an alkaline pH range of 7.35 - 7.45, the range that the body tries to maintain at all times through the process of homeostasis. pH is a term used in chemistry for the amount of acidity or alkalinity of an aqueous solution. The pH scale runs from 0 to 14, with a pH of 7 being neutral, a pH of less than 7 being acidic, and a pH greater than 7 being alkaline.

The basal pH of gastric juices secreted by the glands of the stomach is strongly acidic, with a range of 1.5 - 3.5. The pH in the stomach changes when food is eaten, and is influenced by various psychological factors, including the aroma and taste of foods.

Blood Sampling and Analysis

A blood test is often prescribed by doctors to help diagnose a person's health condition. The blood sample is sent to a laboratory where technicians analyze the blood using specialized instruments and techniques. Various tests may be performed on a blood sample, including a complete blood count (CBC), which is used to detect a wide range of health disorders such as anemia, infection and leukemia, and a blood glucose test, which is used to help diagnose diabetes and monitor blood glucose levels. None of the tests are conclusive in themselves but are used to help diagnose a patient's condition and determine what follow-up tests should be prescribed.

In Appendix D of his book, *The Detox Miracle Sourcebook*, Robert Morse describes how anyone can interpret the results of the blood work that a doctor has prescribed for them. It includes a description of blood types (Types A, B, AB, etc.), the meaning of red and white blood cell counts, and the limitations that the diagnostics have. It lists reference ranges for nutrients that are found in the blood. The ranges are based on analyses of blood of presumably healthy people. But the point is, it seems that the body requires nutrients to be within certain ranges for health.

According to T. Colin Campbell in his book, *Whole, Rethinking the Science of Nutrition,* the body is continually monitoring and adjusting the concentrations of nutrients in the blood to maintain the ranges it requires for health. He explains how medical and governmental understanding of nutrition is rooted in the reductionist paradigm, a way of thinking that everything can be understood through its component parts. He contends that a wholistic approach to health is what is required to understand nutrition.

As explained in the chapter on the Causes of Disease, a wholistic approach considers how the various component parts work together. It considers how they work together in line with how nature operates. Nature works in wholistic ways, with all parts working together, never with one part working on its own.

"When you're looking through a microscope, either literally or metaphorically, you can't see the big picture." - T. Colin Campbell and Howard Jacobson, *Whole, Rethinking the Science of Nutrition.*

An old saying seems to be apropos here, "You can't see the forest for the trees." We cannot see the forest when we are focusing on the trees.

Nutritionists have known for many years that the condition of the urine reveals much about the blood's condition. For example, if the urine is cloudy, the blood is likely to be cloudy too, such as when protein intake has thickened it. The pH of urine closely

The Only Cure for Constipation

matches the pH of the blood, and can be used to determine the blood's pH condition. Litmus paper is a useful tool in this regard. It is another example of how we can become more our own doctor. We can test our urine's pH. Strips of litmus paper may be purchased on the Web.

Chapter 20 Antioxidants

Antioxidants are substances that protect the cells of the body against the effects of free radicals. They include beta-carotene, lycopene, p-coumaric acid, and vitamins A, C, and E (alpha-tocopherol), all of which are found in whole (raw) plant foods. Antioxidants neutralize free radicals.

Free Radicals

A free radical is a molecule that has an unpaired electron. It is "free" to react "radically" with other molecules and cause cellular disruption and damage.

According to the National Cancer Institute, damage to the cells of the body caused by free radicals plays an important role in the development of cancer and other serious health disorders.

Antioxidants are the body's main defenses against free radicals. They neutralize free radicals by chemically combining them with the molecules in the foods. As discussed in the chapter on The Causes of Disease, foods that are rich in antioxidants are known to stop or reverse toxic buildup.

We should eat foods that are high in antioxidants. The foods of a whole plant food diet are rich in enzymes, nutrients and antioxidants. Whole plant foods that are particularly rich in antioxidants are listed below.

WHOLE PLANT FOODS HIGH IN ANTIOXIDANTS

Fruits – all kinds
Green leafy vegetables (Greens) – all kinds

The Only Cure for Constipation

Vegetables – all kinds
Spices and herbs
Superfoods

It is important to eat as many antioxidant-rich foods as we can to strengthen the immune system, neutralize the poisons within the body and stop or reverse toxic buildup in the body.

Most antioxidants are destroyed by heat. While freezing seems to preserve antioxidant activity, heating adversely affects almost all antioxidants. This means, for example, that canned and jarred fruits and vegetables, which have been heat treated during refining and processing, have significantly lower levels of antioxidants than their living food counterparts. It indicates that fruits and vegetables that are fast-frozen are acceptable to eat on a whole plant food diet.

Oxidative Stress

Oxidative stress occurs when an imbalance exists between free radical activity and antioxidant activity in the body. An ordinary diet, such as the Standard American Diet, causes oxidative stress which contributes to aging and degenerative diseases. It is known that when foods contain insufficient antioxidants to counteract free radicals, the resulting imbalance can damage the DNA and the proteins and fatty tissues of the body.

Researchers have shown that mental stress creates free radicals. Radiation, environmental pollutants, such as smog, cigarette smoke, car exhaust fumes and impurities and toxins in municipal drinking water, also create free radicals.

Agricultural chemicals are known to destroy the antioxidants in crops. Therefore, it is wise to eat organic produce to maximize the antioxidants we receive from natural plant foods.

According to Dr. Michael Greger's book, *How Not To Die*, antioxidant supplements, such as vitamin C and beta carotene, do not work. The body needs to get its antioxidants from living plant foods. By eating fruits and vegetables rich in beta carotene you can keep your immune system as well as the rest of your body healthy and happy. The fruits and vegetables that are high in beta carotene include tomatoes, apricots, mangoes, carrots, cabbage, broccoli, cantaloupe, green leaf lettuce, kale, mustard greens, pumpkin, red leaf lettuce, spinach, sweet potatoes, turnip greens and winter squash.

Antioxidant Ratings

The ORAC (Oxygen Radical Absorbance Capacity) is considered a useful antioxidant rating system, although it is not the only one.

ORAC was used by the USDA until 2012, which, according to the Web, was the year USDA's Nutrient Data Laboratory (NDL) removed the ORAC Database for Selected Foods from the NDL website. It was removed due to pressure on the USDA from independent laboratories that argued that "in vitro" tests do not conclusively reflect what happens in the human body. It is uncertain whether the pressure was due to legitimate concerns or based on the biased opinion of the meat and dairy industries. However, it appears to be a somewhat specious argument since measuring the effect of antioxidants in the human body (in vitro) is not possible, according to papers published on the Web at the time of this writing.

The Only Cure for Constipation

Nevertheless, ORAC is still used by many nutritionists as a comparative basis for antioxidant capacity since it reflects how effectively a food or product neutralizes free radicals as measured by the degradation of a fluorescent dye. ORAC is a particularly useful measure of the antioxidant effectiveness of foods that contain complex ingredients with both slow- and fast-acting antioxidants, and also foods that have combined or synergistic effects.

ORAC ratings of various herbs and spices, taken from the Web at the time of this writing, are listed below for comparison purposes.

SAMPLE OF ORAC ANTIOXIDANT RATINGS

Cloves, ground	314, 446
Cinnamon, ground	267, 536
Oregano, dried	200,129
Rosemary, dried	165, 280
Parsley, dried	73, 670

Many foods that are commonly eaten today, such as meat- and dairy-based foods, have, in comparison to the above values, negligible ORAC ratings, which indicates low antioxidant effectiveness. These foods include, but are not limited to, salmon with an ORAC rating of 30, eggs (20), hot dogs (300), McDonald's Crispy Chicken Sandwich (180), Little Caesar's Cheese Pizza (180), and fried chicken (50).

At the time of this writing, a complete listing of ORAC ratings of many foods is available on the following website:

The Only Cure for Constipation

https://www.superfoodly.com/orac-values/.

It should be noted that the ORAC rating is based on 100 grams of food. Since raw fruits and vegetables, including fresh (undried) herbs, have water content, the ORAC ratings of these foods are much lower than their dried alternatives. If this is not considered, the ORAC ratings of raw fruits and vegetables can be misleading.

When we eat living plant foods, the body is provided with all the nutrients it needs for optimum health, including Nature's own antioxidants. The body's defenses against free radicals are the greatest when we eat raw plant foods, which means the immune system is strengthened by these foods. Antioxidant supplements, such as the vitamin C and beta carotene supplements that are available today, are not good sources for the antioxidants the body needs. A whole plant food diet is the best assurance that anyone can have of getting the antioxidants needed for health.

Chapter 21 The Foods We Should Eat and Why

Increasing scientific evidence compiled every year links the nominal top 10 leading causes of death, and the degenerative diseases so prevalent in the world today, to eating meat-based and dairy-based diets. These studies continue to show that people eating a plant-based diet have increased longevity and health compared to those eating a meat-based and/or dairy-based diet. Many books published in recent years provide the results of these clinical studies.

The China Study, published in 2005, may be the most comprehensive study of human nutrition ever performed. The population, or group, that was used in the study was the entire population of China. Written by T. Colin Campbell, a professor of Nutritional Biochemistry at Cornell University, and his son Thomas M. Campbell II, a physician, the study proved that whole plant-based foods, not animal-based foods, are the most beneficial foods for people. The study showed that people eating a plant-based diet have increased longevity and health compared to those eating a meat-based and/or dairy-based diet.

How Not to Die, written by Dr. Michael Greger and published in 2015, confirmed the conclusions of *The China Study*, and provided additional research and study results that emphasized the importance of eating plenty of whole plant foods, such as fruits and vegetables, to prevent and even reverse the chronic diseases of the Western world, including cancer, diabetes, heart disease and brain diseases.

The hazards of eating animal-based foods, or animal products, are well known to most educated people. Eating animal products causes plaque formations in the arteries, which is known to cause hardening of the arteries, which can lead to heart disease and stroke. Harmful mutagens and carcinogens, such as acrylamide, HCAs, PAHs and AGEs, are formed when animal products are cooked (for more detail, see Victoria Boutenko's book, *12 Steps to Raw Foods*). Animal products can contain nitrates, chlorine and ammonia and are susceptible to hosting various forms of life-destroying bacteria.

Studies conducted on animals and people show that blood cholesterol levels increase when animal protein is eaten. Dr. Caldwell Esselstyn, Jr., in his book, *Prevent and Reverse Heart Disease*, says that anyone with high blood cholesterol levels is prone to heart disease. Animal-based foods contain cholesterol, whereas no plant foods contain cholesterol. Dr. Esselstyn changed his diet to a plant-based diet and strongly recommended his patients to do the same. Those who did were able to cleanse their coronary arteries of plaque formations, which means their arteries were no longer clogged, and Dr. Esselstyn proved this by way of coronary angiograms.

Dr. Esselstyn is now a leading advocate of raw plant foods. He is featured in the food documentary DVD, *Forks Over Knives*. Testimonies given in that DVD attest to the powers of raw plant foods to heal a number of leading chronic diseases, including heart disease and breast cancer.

High blood cholesterol can also cause brain diseases, because excess cholesterol in the blood can lead to excess cholesterol in the brain. Autopsies have revealed that Alzheimer's brains have significantly more cholesterol build up than normal brains.[301]

In *Fruits and Farinacea – The Proper Food of Man*, John Smith tells us that based on all accessible sources, our progenitors were frugivorous, i.e., fruit eaters. Both anthropological studies and studies of how the human body functions support this conclusion.

"Meat is not man's natural food, since he is not either a carnivorous or an omnivorous animal. Every argument drawn from comparative anatomy, from physiology, from chemistry, from experience, from observation, and, when rightly used, from common sense, all agree that man is not a meat-eating animal. He can never be as healthy under the prevailing "mixed" diet as he would if he were to follow the dictates of Nature and live on his natural food – fruits and nuts, eaten in their uncooked, primitive form. Every element the system needs can be shown to be present in these foods, in their proper proportion, while, being live foods instead of mere "dead ashes", which is all the cooking process leaves, they will be found to supply a degree of vital life and energy which no cooked foods ever supplied or could supply."
- Hereward Carrington, *Vitality, Fasting and Nutrition*.

Human beings, in many key physiological ways, are not like other animals. We have hands with opposable thumbs, non-claw-like nails, teeth that are not suitable for tearing hide or flesh, or breaking bones, but rather for grinding plant foods, and long, not short, digestive tracts including 20-25 foot long intestines that are ideally suited for digesting fiber-rich foods like fruits, vegetables, nuts, seeds and grains.

David Wolfe in his book, *The Sunfood Diet Success System*,

---

[301] Dr. Michael Greger, How Not To Die,

The Only Cure for Constipation

includes as Appendix A, an "Anatomy Chart" that identifies 17 physiological ways in which human beings are ideally suited for eating a plant-based diet. Websites also support this conclusion, as can be seen by searching on "Are humans frugivores?"

These studies show that humans are naturally suited for picking, chewing and digesting plant-based foods. Chimpanzees, which are very similar to humans physiologically, subsist almost entirely on fruits and greens.

According to the Bible, the first people on earth lived to very great ages. Adam lived to 930 years   Methuselah lived 969 years. Prior to the Flood, the average human lifespan was about 900 years. However, immediately after the Flood, when animal food was permitted to be eaten, the average lifespan fell to about 400 years. Later, when Jacob, the father of the twelve tribes of Israel, lived, the average lifespan was only about 150 years.

Based on the latest worldwide statistics from WHO, the average human lifespan is 72 years.

Scientists tell us that the human brain has billions of cells but no more than a tenth of them are ever used. It would make sense if the brain, as well as the rest of the human organism, was designed to last for hundreds of years instead of less than a hundred.

The worldwide increase in food production has resulted in a worldwide topsoil mineral deficiency. The topsoil in which plants are grown is now depleted of its minerals. Reports on the Web cover recent losses of nutrients in crops. Only decades ago, the same crops were richer in vitamins and minerals. Meat and dairy products (animal products) are affected even worse. Animals consume the mineral deficient crops and become mineral deficient. Cooking animal products further depletes them of minerals and vitamins.

The mineral deficiency of the topsoil is being blamed on improper farm management practices resulting in ill-replenishment of the minerals back into the soil. The meteoric rise in food productivity and efficiency since the last century have not been balanced by a corresponding increase in the addition of nutrients back into the soil.

Nutritional deficiency occurs when the body does not absorb or get enough of the necessary amounts of nutrients it needs from foods. Nutrients include vitamins, minerals, proteins, carbohydrates, fats and water. They are essential for cellular growth and the maintenance of life. The body does not manufacture nutrients, but obtains them from the surrounding environment. We get most of our nutrients from foods.

People who eat the traditional American diet are nutrient deficient. This deficiency has been shown to be the cause of a number of serious health problems. To make up for the mineral-starved and vitamin-starved foods now being produced, many people take multivitamin/mineral supplements on the advice of their doctors. According to the Web, billions of dollars are spent each year in America alone on these supplements.

Unfortunately, most of the multivitamin/mineral supplements are inorganic substances that cannot be utilized by the body. Studies have shown that these supplements provide little, if any, benefit to human health. See Web articles, such as from searching on "multivitamin/mineral supplements." It is also discussed in books by Dr. Ann Wigmore (see Bibliography), among others.

The Only Cure for Constipation

"Inorganic minerals are rejected by the cells of the body, which, if not evacuated, can cause arterial obstructions and even more serious damage." - Norman W. Walker, *Water Can Undermine Your Health*.

According to many nutritionists who are referenced in this book, the cells of the body can only utilize minerals that are in organic form, which is one of the reasons why plant foods are so important to us. Plants convert inorganic minerals found in the soil and water into organic form that is readily assimilated by the cells of the body.

Doctors often prescribe medication that is calcium carbonate based, which is an inorganic mineral compound. Calcium carbonate is the main ingredient in almost all antacids, and it is also found in some brands of Aspirin.

The days when milk cows roamed the pastures and got their calcium from grass are over. Today's milk cows do not go outside to graze. They seldom move out of their stalls or feedlots. Their urine and feces are removed mechanically. Their milk is removed by machines hooked up to their udders. They get their calcium and other nutrients from their feed, which, according to Web articles, is a specially formulated mix of grains, soy, silage and inorganic calcium in the form of calcite flour (calcium carbonate), aragonite (calcium carbonate), crushed bones, and other bits and pieces of slaughtered animals to maximize weight gain and therefore profits when the cows are no longer useful as money-making machines. Apparently, calcium from cow's milk is mainly inorganic calcium.

On a whole plant food diet, there is no need for multivitamin/mineral supplements, since all the minerals and vitamins needed to support life are in raw plant foods in their proper organic form and undestroyed by heat. An example is the amount of organic calcium that is in collard greens. According to the USDA publication Nutritive Value of American Foods, just two-thirds cup of collard greens has 91% of the calcium in a cup of milk. Other plant foods having about the same amount of calcium are kelp and almonds.

A whole plant food diet also compensates for topsoil mineral deficiency since more plant foods are eaten on the diet. In addition, the diet includes sea vegetables, which are grown in the ocean – a mineral-rich environment.

Nutritional deficiency is so widespread in this country and in the world today that it can be said to be the number one health problem in the world, even among people who supposedly eat a healthy, balanced diet.

Excitotoxins are substances added to processed foods and beverages for the purpose of stimulating brain neurons. For years, the food industry has designed food products to titillate the taste buds and activate the reward centers of the brain. The diverse chemicals that are used for these purposes include excitotoxins. The term was popularized by Dr. Russel Blaylock in his book, *Excitotoxins, The Taste that Kills*. As stated in the book, these substances are found in almost all processed foods. Excitotoxins include monosodium glutamate (MSG)[302], aspartame (used in artificial sweeteners), cysteine (used in breads), hydrolyzed protein, and aspartic acid. These substances can

---

[302] According to Blaylock's book, the food industry is on a quest to disguise MSG in foods. A list of common additives that contain MSG is found in the book.

stimulate brain neurons so severely that they are killed, resulting in varying degrees of brain damage.

Remember that piercing headache you got the last time you ate Chinese food? It was probably due to the MSG used on the food. The Web adequately covers the dangers of MSG, e.g., do a search on "msg in foods."

As of this writing, there are no regulations requiring the food industry to test its products for whether they cause brain damage or food addictions.

The deliberate tampering of foods to increase taste appeal at the expense of harming the body, while attesting to the inventiveness and ingenuity of the American spirit, typifies how low we have sunk in manipulating foods for financial gain.

It is entirely possible that the causative factor, or at least a major contributing factor, to the sharp rise in brain diseases in our culture, including dementia and other neurological disorders, is the continued use year after year of food products that contain excitotoxins. I recommend Dr. Baylock's book to anyone. It includes a list of chemicals that should be tacked to our kitchen walls. It will make you check the foods labels all over again.

To avoid the hazards that have been described, and more (I'm sure I haven't mentioned all of them) we should eat raw plant foods. This is what nutritional experts have been telling us for years, as documented in their books listed in the Bibliography.

We live in the age of information, and the Web/Internet is our most popular information source. While I consider the Web a very useful tool for learning about foods and nutrition, it should not be our only source for this information. Much of what is on websites is opinion-oriented or provided in support of commercial interests. Opinions can run the gamut, and misrepresentation and conflicting information can be, and often times are, the result.

"As corrupting an influence as money is in medicine, it appears to be even worse in the field of nutrition, where it seems everyone has his or her own brand of snake oil supplement or wonder gadget. Dogmas are entrenched and data too often cherry picked to support preconceived notions." - Dr. Michael Greger, *How Not To Die*.

For example, for years leading nutritionists have contended that cooked and starchy foods are detrimental to human health, and that abstinence from such foods is necessary to cure health disorders including diseases. However, at the time of this writing, many websites queried for this information actually encourage eating cooked and starchy foods as part of a healthy diet.

We cannot trust everything we read on the Web. But that being said, the Web should not be ignored as a learning tool in self-education about foods and nutrition. However, for those of us who are seeking answers to the really tough questions of today about foods and nutrition, books provide the answers. The books that are listed in the Bibliography are excellent resources that will aid anyone in their quest for a more thorough understanding of foods and nutrition.

Books have the answers on how to gain optimum health, the Web does not. Books cannot be easily condensed into Web articles, and typically provide comprehensive coverage of the issues, or they refer to other books or studies that provide the information. In addition, books are typically written by competent and knowledgeable authors who provide good, proven advice.

The Only Cure for Constipation

Today's real need is not another low-carb, high-protein diet, or an end to global warming, which appears to be mainly caused by extensive deforestation efforts to clear space for cattle and feed crops.[303] Rather, it is self-education about foods and nutrition.

Typically, people resort to doctors when they don't know what else to do. But by simply utilizing the Web/Internet, as well as the information that is contained in books that are available to most people, many health concerns can be thoroughly investigated, and the proper treatments determined, without seeing a physician.

The body can take a lot of punishment and abuse. It can survive both drought and famine. It can live on junk food for decades without showing many ill effects. But the body does not thrive on drought or famine or junk food. It thrives on life-giving plant foods. If optimum health is the goal, then a change in the diet is required.

None of us has to die of a disease caused by a bad diet, and none of us has to suffer the many complications and discomforts that a disease entails. And we won't, if we take care of our bodies by giving it the life-giving and sustaining foods it needs.

As stated previously, it is our responsibility to take care of our bodies. It is not our doctor's, our spouse's, our friends' or the Government's. It is our responsibility. We should avoid foods that are harmful to health and eat foods that promote health and longevity. These are whole plant foods, replete with their life-giving properties. These are the foods that God and Nature intended for us to eat.

Fruits and Vegetables

---

[303] www.nature.com/scitable/blog/green-science/deforestation_and_global.

The Only Cure for Constipation

Raw fruits and vegetables should be eaten regularly. They digest efficiently because their enzymes have not been destroyed by heat.

As discussed in detail in the chapter on Dangers to Avoid, enzymes have life force properties that Nature intended for us to receive, that support all bodily functions and contain the vitamins and nutrients the body needs for optimum health.

Fruits and vegetables are best eaten when they are ripe. If eaten in their typical store-bought, un-ripened condition, stomachache or some other discomfort is likely. Also, extra energy is required to digest them, and this energy is taken from the energy reserves of the body when it could be used for other purposes, such as healing and self-cleansing.

Fruits and vegetables sold at local food stores are typically shipped-in from distant locations, such as foreign countries, and purposely arrive in an un-ripened condition in order to retard spoilage and prolong shelf-life. To ripen store-bought fruits and vegetables, just set them on the counter tops at home until they are ripe; it usually takes several days, depending on the fruit or vegetable. For example, bananas are typically sold green or partly green in color, unless you happen by the fruit stand right before the bananas are replaced. Ripe bananas are speckled or streaked brown in color, which typically takes several days.

Cucumbers are ripe when they are easily flexed. Avocados are ripe when they yield to gentle pressure. Green chilies and jalapenos are ripe when they turn orange or red; do not eat them when they are green. Lemons, limes, oranges and pears are ripe when they are aromatic. Same for red and yellow peppers.

The Only Cure for Constipation

Some exceptions to this are apples (all varieties) and root vegetables (e.g., carrots, beets, turnips, radishes, potatoes, onions, garlic, etc.). Apples and root vegetables do not ripen to any significant extent after they are picked.

Fruits are nutritious and stimulating, and have many healing qualities. They act to cleanse and energize the cells of the body. I consider fruits to be the ideal food for humankind, and we are blessed indeed to have such a plenteous supply.

"Fruits alone, even of but one kind, not only heal but nourish perfectly the human body, eliminating entirely the possibility of disease." - Arnold Ehret, *Mucusless Diet Healing System*.

Some people will not eat fruit because the last time they did, it caused them too much discomfort. Most likely, it was because the fruit was eaten in an un-ripened condition, or else it was combined improperly with other foods. For example, when dates or figs are eaten with pineapple, the result may be a stomachache, because, as discussed in the chapter on The Proper Food Combinations, sweet fruit (dates and figs) should not be eaten with acid fruit (pineapple).

Fatty fruits include avocados and olives. They contain healthy unsaturated fat. Some nutritional experts consider avocado a Superfood, although it is not classified as such. The avocado contains a substantial amount of monounsaturated fats, phytosterols and antioxidants like vitamin E, vitamin C, and carotenoids. It is also high in beta-sitosterol (95 mg per medium-sized avocado) which is known to assist in relieving prostate disorders, such as benign prostatic hyperplasia (BPH).

The vegetables that have the most tightly compacted layers are some of the most nutritious. They include red and green cabbage, leeks, broccoli, bok choy, green onions, lettuce and celery.

Carrots are high in beta-carotene which is converted to vitamin A in the body. The word "carotene" is derived from the Latin word for carrot, "carota." Nutritional expert N.W. Walker in his books states that raw carrots have all the elements and vitamins that are required by the human body. It could just be that the "lowly carrot" is capable of making up for many of the nutritional deficiencies in the world today.

Carrots are non-starchy vegetables as explained in the chapter on Proper Food Combinations.

Red beets are good for the blood. They lower blood pressure. They improve athletic performance. They are one of the highest of oxygenating foods. Marathon runners are partial to them because they increase their endurance. After consuming red beets, it takes less energy to run a race. This makes red beets important for elderly health, since studies have shown that there is a decline in maximal oxygen consumption with age (unless you do aerobics). In addition, red beets have a high acid-binding rating as seen in Berg's Tables in Appendix I.

Leafy greens are commonly considered vegetables. They include spinach, arugula, chard, kale (several varieties), mustard greens, collard greens, turnip greens, parsley, cilantro, lettuce (several varieties), celery greens and dandelion. The chlorophyll in greens strengthens the immune system, helps to detoxify the body and improves digestion. Chlorophyll is rich in antioxidants, minerals, vitamins and readily assimilated enzymes. The chlorophyll in green plants is what converts sunlight into chemical energy, and this energy is made available to us when we eat greens.

The Only Cure for Constipation

No fruit or vegetable is intrinsically better than another. Each may be preferred, or not, depending on a person's nutritional needs and personal preferences. We all have grown to like certain fruits or vegetables better than others, and we all have slightly different nutritional needs. The only way to learn what fruits and vegetables are best for us, is to eat a variety of them in their ripened states, and, if not by themselves in mono meals, then ensuring that they are eaten properly combined with other foods.

David Wolfe states in one of his books that there are so many edible fruits and vegetables in the world that if you tried a new kind every day of your life, you would never live long enough to try them all. So, what is stopping us from trying the 40-50 varieties of fruits and vegetables that are in our local food stores? It's the only way to know whether they work for us nutritionally and otherwise.

Grains and Legumes

Technically speaking, grains are seeds of grasses. However, they are commonly considered to be vegetables. Grains include wheat, corn, oats, barley, rye, millet, and rice. Grain products include refined flour products, such as all breads (white, whole wheat, rye, etc.), oats, cereal, white and brown rice and pasta.

As discussed previously, grains are starchy foods and acid-forming foods, and a main contributor to constipation. Their high acid-forming scores can be seen in Berg's Tables in Appendix I. Starch is gooey and pasty. As stated before, it is used for glues and hanging wallpaper. It sticks to the walls of the lower intestine and causes all kinds of problems, as discussed in the chapter on The Causes of Disease and the chapter on Dangers to Avoid.

"At least 90% of the 'diet of civilization' contains these sticky foods and man stuffs himself daily with awful mixtures of them. Thus the digestive tract ids not only clogged up through constipation, but literally glued together with sticky mucus and feces." Arnold Ehret, *The Definite Cure of Chronic Constipation.*

Legumes include peas, beans, peanuts and lentils. Legumes are commonly considered to be vegetables. Like grains, they are starchy foods, and for that reason I no longer eat them, with the exception of sweet corn, as discussed in the chapter on What Everyone Should Know About Fiber, nor do I advise their use.

A healthy diet is one that is low in saturated fats and Omega-6 oils, and high in natural fiber, vitamins, minerals and other nutrients found in whole plant foods as opposed to supplements or man-made foods   According to the government's Dietary Guidelines for Americans, people should get most of their nutrients from food and beverages rather than supplements.[304]

Proper Eating Habits

"We are not what we eat but what we assimilate" - Paavo O. Airola.

Those who wolf, gulp or bolt down their foods are prone to digestive discomforts and disorders, including heartburn and stomachache to mention only two. Many regularly resort to quick remedies, such as antacids, Aspirin and similar drugs. According to the Web, at least $2 billion are spent yearly in the US alone on antacids, and $10 billion worldwide. That's a lot of indigestion!

In addition, many people eat compulsively, often consuming food throughout the day whenever they feel like it, whether they're hungry or not. Compulsive eating can be out of habit or because

---

[304] https://ods.od.nih.gov/factsheets/Magnesium-Consumer/.

of job-prescribed or tradition-prescribed meal times. If we eat food when we are not hungry, the body is not ready for the food.

These habits are damaging to the human system, and the damage gets worse the more they are practiced. They cannot produce vibrant health because the foods cannot be properly digested and assimilated by the body. Not only do they cause digestive difficulties and constipation, but they cause sluggishness and grogginess, general fatigue and various illnesses.

Again, the old saying:

One quarter of what you eat keeps you alive. The other quarter keeps your doctor alive.

Proper eating habits are prescribed by Nature. Food must be eaten in such a way that the full powers of the digestive system are employed. In addition, every ounce of food that passes through the body that is not actually needed by the body is a tax on the body's vital powers, a waste of vital energy.

To avoid these complications and more, most of us need to modify our eating habits.

As stated in the chapter on The Digestive System, digestion is a chemical process assisted by chewing that breaks down food into constituents that can be assimilated by the body. It breaks down carbohydrates, fats and proteins (macronutrients) into smaller components that can be utilized by the cells of the body for energy, maintenance, growth and repair.

Food intake activates the digestive system. Food activates the secretion of saliva in the mouth as it does digestive, or gastric, juices in the stomach where the juices further breakdown the food.

The Only Cure for Constipation

The job of digestion is not finished until the food travels through the small and large intestines and the waste passes out of the body.

Mechanical digestion occurs as the teeth grind and masticate food. Chewing breaks down food into smaller particles which allows them to be better digested. An old saying is: "Chew your food, your stomach has no teeth."

As discussed in the chapter on The Digestive System, chemical digestion begins in the mouth through saliva. If the mouth does not water during a meal, then the body is not ready for the food, and digestion of that food will be hindered. Some nutritionists claim that well-salivated food is practically half-digested before it gets to the stomach. Many raw foodists recommend chewing food until it is liquified in the mouth. In addition, whenever whole plant foods are eaten, the enzymes in these foods assist in the chemical digestive process. Otherwise, the enzyme reserves in the body must be used.

Two thousand years ago, Asclepiades of Greece understood that particles of food are a main cause of indigestion. If the particles were small, digestion would follow its normal course, but if the particles were too big, indigestion would occur.

"The chief function of today's cook is to prepare soft pap for the adult, so that little or no chewing is required. Meats are pounded or ground and vegetables cooked to make them easy to swallow with a minimum of chewing; breads are made to be swallowed with very little preliminary mastication; potatoes are mashed, cereals soaked and fruits stewed, so that the muscles of the jaw get very little exercise and the food gets very little saliva. There is no real pleasure in such eating." - Dr. Herbert M. Shelton, *Health for the Millions*.

The Only Cure for Constipation

To get the most of foods, and produce the kind of health we all want and need, the following eating habits should be practiced at every meal.

1. All foods should be eaten slowly, and chewed thoroughly. If you are very hungry before eating, you should still slow down on the eating or the foods will be wolfed or bolted down with little chewing taking place.

2. Do not overeat. This is the cardinal rule to master if you want to obtain optimum health. The best advice I can offer is the same as that of many others, which is to leave the table when you are 2/3 full. This has often been difficult for me to learn, for as the old saying goes, "our eyes are bigger than our stomachs," but I found that when I practiced it everything changed for the better on my journey to optimum health. It amounts to eating only as much as your system actually needs. Only you can determine that. It may take a while to get right, but it is all part of the journey.

To lengthen your life, shorten your meals.

"Every individual should, as a general rule, restrain himself to the smallest quantity which he finds from careful investigation, enlightened experience and observation will fully meet the alimentary wants of his system, knowing that whatsoever is more than this is evil." - Dr. Sylvester Graham.

I believe that most people who are striving for optimum health soon begin to eat less food, not because they feel differently about eating, necessarily, but because they realize from the clues the body gives them that they really don't *need* much food, and probably never did.

Not everyone has the same proclivity, or liking, for foods, or the same nutritional requirements. But the body requires similar things for health and wellness, and we are all very much alike in numerous ways, having the same basic needs, the same general physiology, the same susceptibility to biological disharmony, the same susceptibility to many illnesses, and we share many of the same stresses, worries and fears that can influence our state of health. Nutritionists, whose voices have not been heard as much as those of ordinary diet proponents, have been telling us for years that ill health and diseases of all types spring most often from one common source, namely, poor dietary practices.

3. Adhere to the proper food combination laws as discussed in the chapter on Proper Food Combinations.

4. Make sure fruits are ripe before eating them. How to tell when fruits are ready to be eaten was discussed previously.

5. Enjoy your food! If food is not enjoyed it cannot be efficiently digested.

6. If emotionally strung out or upset about something before eating, then skip the meal. Studies have shown that fear, anxiety, tension and anger constrict the entire digestive system and dry up the digestive juices.

7. Limit water or other fluid intake during a meal. It only dilutes the digestive juices that are needed for proper digestion. Drink liquids at least 1/2 hour before, and typically no sooner than 1 hour after a meal. Protein and fat meals require the longest times to pass through the stomach (up to 4 hours), so adjust the consumption of liquids after the meal accordingly.

8. The simplest meals are the best. Get into the habit of eating simple meals consisting of salads with fresh and ripe vegetables.

Chapter 22 The Food Pyramid

The United States Department of Agriculture (USDA) has issued its Food Guide Pyramid since 1992. The Guide is intended to help Americans reduce their intake of total fat and choose what and how much to eat from each of the food groups that are depicted on the pyramid. The government's involvement in the issuance of nutritional guidelines shows how far we have drifted away from the basics of proper health and nutrition.

The food pyramid is often displayed on packaged foods, such as breads. However, it is the firm conviction of many nutritionists that the USDA Food Pyramid does not, and never has, properly reflected what is best for human health. Rather, it reflects what the food industry says is best for health.

The meat, dairy and grain businesses, which are the chief vested interests in perpetuating the Standard American Diet, have influenced federal dietary regulations for decades. It is commonly believed that these interests write the protocols of the USDA. As stated in a dietary guideline article published on the Web, "After all, what is the USDA if not the regulatory body created to ensure that the U.S. agricultural commodities (like corn, soy, and wheat) are profitable?" These interests are interested first, last and always in profits, not in human welfare.

It is well known that most of the grain produced in the world goes to feed livestock in order to supply food stores and restaurants with cold cuts and other meat products.

Most of us realize by now the power that big businesses have to make the rules. But health awareness and a knowledge of foods and nutrition give us the freedom to eat the healthier foods that are available for us to eat.

The food pyramid is not our friend. When I started searching for the answers about how foods and nutrition impact human health years ago, I was often led astray by the food pyramid because of my gullibility to accept what governmental bodies recommend should be my diet. As discussed in this book, many nutritionists, including those whose books are listed in the Bibliography, have been telling us for years that meat, dairy and grain products are harmful to human health.

The food pyramid of 1992 to 2005 (see below) shows bread, cereal, rice and pasta at the bottom, or base, of the pyramid, indicating that grain products should be the most often eaten food. However, all grains, even raw grain seeds, are starchy foods. And pasta, sweet rolls and bread are cooked foods. As discussed in this book, cooked and starchy foods are harmful to human health. For a healthy diet, the food pyramid would not have grain products as the base, nor would it include cooked foods.

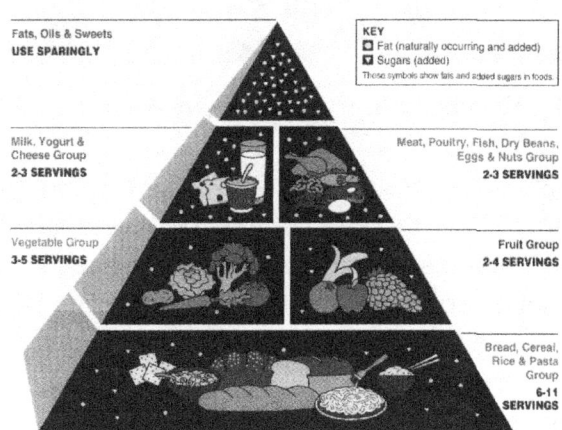

The Food Guide Pyramid from 1992 to 2005

The Only Cure for Constipation

With all the food that is available to us, I think we can be a little more particular.

The food pyramid of 2005 to 2011 (below), makes even less sense. It doesn't have a clearly defined base or hierarchy. It shows five food groups (grains, vegetables, fruits, milk, and meat and beans), sharing the same base. There is no one food group at the base of the pyramid. At first glance, it indicates that there is no one food group any better for health than another. It implies that you should eat a portion of each.

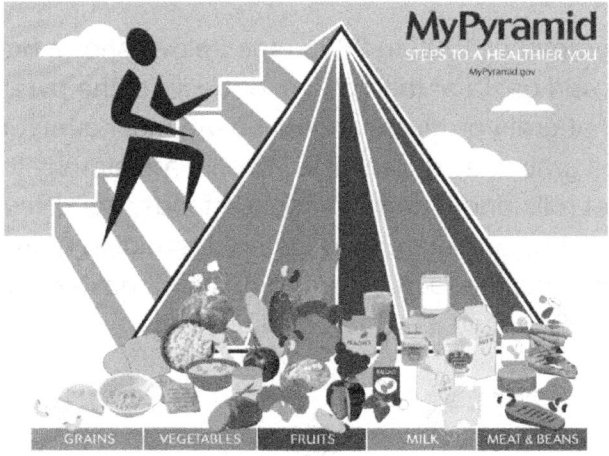

The Food Guide Pyramid from 2005 to 2011

It is not surprising that grains, milk and meat are three of the five food groups that share the base of this food pyramid. The meat, dairy and grain businesses are those with the largest vested interests in continuing the production of animal products for the Standard American Diet.

For most of us, the food pyramid of 2005 to 2011 is too confusing to be an effective dietary guideline.

The Only Cure for Constipation

The Food Pyramid has recently (2019) been superseded by MyPlate (see below), also published by the USDA. MyPlate is a depiction of a pie-shaped plate of food on a table with a drink off to one side. Five food groups, Fruits, Vegetables, Grains, Proteins and Milk, are represented.

There are no MyPlate details in the depiction to reveal what each food group consists of, but they may be accessed on the Web. For example, for Fruits, the details list as options, fresh, canned, frozen, dried, cut up or pureed. For Proteins, the details list seafood, meat, poultry and eggs, nuts, seeds and soy. The drink off to the side is milk. The dangers of eating canned food products, and most of the protein options (excepting nuts and seeds), have been discussed in this book. Also, as discussed previously, vegetables provide all the proteins needed for human health. The MyPlate design implies that we need to eat foods from all five food groups, including dairy, and in every form sold to the public.

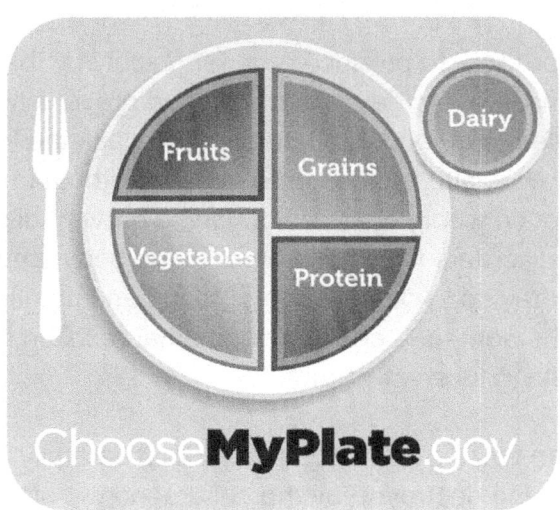

The current (2019) USDA Food Guideline

The Only Cure for Constipation

In the age of information, a food pyramid or pie plate that would really make sense would be one that would give priority to eating raw fruits and vegetables over everything else, with nuts, seeds, and water included in the design. It would not include meat- and dairy-based foods, grain products or canned foods.

However, it probably doesn't matter what the food pyramids or other depictions look like. Guidelines do not make people knowledgeable no matter how instructive they may be. Knowledge about foods and nutrition is not gained by glancing at a food pyramid or pie chart. Our current obesity epidemic, as described in Chapter 16, clearly indicates the public's failure to follow any dietary guidelines.

People make society what it is. Most people eat whatever they want as often as they want, regardless of the complications and discomforts that result. But what most people eat and how they eat does not have to be the way that we eat.

Each of us can work to produce a better society by the food choices we make every day. As mentioned previously, unless we have a knowledge of foods and nutrition, we lack the information needed on how health issues come about. Without this knowledge, we remain wholly ignorant of how to prevent diseases and other health disorders from taking root in the body, and how to cure them if they do. A knowledge of foods and nutrition enables us to make the right food choices, those that result in real health, which is health in tune with Nature.

We must learn what is best for us to eat and carefully guard our health from being destroyed by the cultural norms of the tempting world.

Chapter 23 How Eating Habits Are Formed

I have often found it beneficial to examine the things that are taken for granted, especially when it comes to foods and nutrition.

Whether old or young, male or female, the main criterion for food choices for most people is how foods taste and go down rather than how they affect health. In other words, taste-appeal over health-appeal. Unfortunately, this truth has been exploited by the many concerns of the food industry in the creation of many substances that are added to our foods and drinks to make them more appetizing. The second basis for food selection is the emotional pull that certain foods have on us. These criteria drive the majority of our decisions about foods. They also cause food habits.

Food habits are long-standing patterns of behavior associated with eating. Those of us who grew up on burgers, French fries and soft drinks tend to stick with that menu, or slight variations of it, throughout life, unless of course change is initiated.

It is now evident to most people that many of the health disorders prevalent in this country and throughout the world are diet-related. However, many of us continue to eat just as we did last year and the year before because of our habits. Another reason is that we have been culturally indoctrinated to believe that certain foods, such as meat and dairy products, sugary foods and drinks, and refined and processed foods, are somehow good for us. Both pressures are reducing our numbers rapidly. Eating foods that we grew up on is not working.

A habit once formed and persistently practiced eventually turns into a craving, whether for chocolates, ice cream, sweet rolls or anything else. The worst part of cravings is that they stay with us even when they are doing us harm.

Food cravings are encouraged by the many advertisements in the media for foods and drinks. Despite their oftentimes silky persuasiveness, the products being sold are, for the most part, refined and processed foods and drinks that have been heat treated, chemically altered, devitalized and robbed of precious nutrients. Not surprisingly, many of the ads support the meat, dairy and grain interests, the chief vested interests in our food industry. Are fast-food establishments purveyors of death as some nutritionists contend? It may be more correct to say that they are purveyors of what most people like to eat.

Learning the truth versus hype about foods and nutrition is the best way to reach health goals. The insight and knowledge gained during the learning process is priceless, for very few things are as important as health.

Anyone with a little persistence and willpower can change their eating habits, or for that matter any other habit in life. Voluntary change begins in the mind. Healthy eating habits are formed when we become convinced that dietary change is in our best interests.

However, many people believe that they are, and have been, living healthy lives, and in particular, they believe that they are eating healthy foods, even when they have health issues. But this is belied when the causes of disease and lesser health disorders are examined.

I grew up at the time when fast-food franchises were just starting out in this country. I was hooked on, and for years ate, the foods of the Standard American Diet. But as I learned more and more about foods and nutrition, and saw the ill effects that the diet had on myself and others, I began eating healthier foods.

People in this country should be the healthiest people on earth. It certainly seems that way since there are now more varieties of health promoting and sustaining foods available to us than ever before, and many of them are organically grown. But we are not the healthiest people because of our preferences for artificial, man-made foods and drinks, our giving way to cultural norms and traditions about foods, and our unwillingness, and even refusal, to abide by Nature's laws that govern health and well-being.

By choosing to ignore the information that has been gained in the human health field that proves that diseases and a host of lesser human ailments are caused by commonly eaten foods, many of us are sacrificing our health for eating habits and food cravings.

"Once I had an overwhelming Diet Coke craving and went to the 7-11 and got a Big Gulp. The baby inside me shook for hours afterward. (I did vow never to do that again.) My blood pressure, always about 93/55, rose to 120/80. I gained 65 pounds. My ankles swelled up with edema to the point where, as a trick at parties, I'd push my finger in and watch how the depression in my ankles stayed there for 30 seconds. I developed hemorrhoids and terrible blood sugar problems. I once saw a former boyfriend as I was walking through the mall and said hello, but my face was so fat he just gave me a strange look and kept walking. He had no idea who I was." - Robyn Openshaw, *The Green Smoothies Diet.*

One can forgive oneself up to a certain point for not knowing how significantly foods affect health. However, if you have experienced the quality of a constipation-free life and then subject

The Only Cure for Constipation

yourself once again to the torments of a constipated life, you are guilty of destroying your health.

Robin Openshaw, who was quoted above, and who, like the majority of nutritionists and nutrition-mined medical doctors, learned health the hard way through self-education about foods and nutrition, writes:

"I know which foods are truly nutritious and which aren't. This is information that the vast majority of Americans do not have. It's not just that they lack self-discipline or make poor choices – they truly don't know because of the false and downright injurious education they have received. I know how to heal and build my own body and my children's with nutrition. I know how to cleanse the organs of elimination whenever necessary. Most importantly, I know how to avoid the need for all that, massively reducing our risk of not only degenerative diseases like cancer and heart disease, but also of simple colds and flu, by just eating simply, low on the food chain, every day." - Robyn Openshaw, *The Green Smoothies Diet.*

Chapter 24 Sleep and Constipation

All parts of the body work together; all parts are interconnected. No one part is completely independent of another. For example, the kidneys and the brain are interconnected. If any part is damaged, injured or adversely affected in some way, it can be expected that other parts are adversely affected in some way too. Treating just one or two parts of the body with drugs, such as treating constipation with laxatives, will not reduce the adverse effects of constipation on all body parts, and it could make things worse for, as we have seen, drugs for constipation can affect the proper functioning of other parts of the body.

It only makes sense, then, that constipation would affect sleep. Mind and body are interconnected; they cannot be separated, so what happens to one affects the other. Clogged up intestinal wastes affect our thoughts, and this is seen not only in our conscious thoughts but also in our dreams.

All living things sleep – humans, animals, fish, reptiles, insects, even plants. All require periods of slumber. A law of Nature is the need for adequate rest. But in our fast-paced society with its unrelenting demands on our time and money, our minds cry out for adequate rest. We are told that eight hours of sleep per night are required for health, but many of us get less than five.

Sleep is a state of unconsciousness that helps the body rest, recharge and repair. When sleep is denied or impaired, and especially when continually impaired, we suffer in mind and body. It causes a sleep deficit, which many people never make up.

Loss of sleep can occur for many reasons, but usually it occurs when we are worried about something that happened or did not

The Only Cure for Constipation

happen, or that might happen. It can disturb sleep. But the foods we eat and how they are digested also can disturb sleep.

Eating foods that are difficult to digest and don't go well with the system causes gastrointestinal problems as previously explained, including but not limited to indigestion, gas and constipation. They arise typically because of what was eaten during the day, the day before, or the day before that. While most people accept them as normal, none of them is normal, and none of them has to occur.

Eating too much salty foods before going to bed can also disrupt sleep. It causes blood pressure to rise, which makes it harder to get to sleep and sleep peacefully. It can also cause itching that can keep one awake.

An important characteristic of the mineral potassium is that it helps the kidneys flush out excess sodium (salt) from the body. Eating foods that are rich in potassium, such as avocado, potatoes, red beets and bananas, during the day can reduce high blood pressure and help a person sleep. For more information, see the book, *How to Cure High Blood Pressure*, listed in the Bibliography.

The frustrations of the day can cut into dreamtime and cause dreams to be repetitive or not make any sense. Often they're meaningless dreams, totally unlike those that make us feel refreshed the morning after. Want good sleeps? Reduce the amount of stress in your life and cure constipation.

"The best cure for the body is a quiet mind." - Napoleon Bonaparte.

Because constipation is dehydrating, it is often accompanied by dried up nasal passages that can disrupt sleep. It can be because we did not drink enough fluids during the day and/or because of the drugs we take that dehydrate the body.

For sound sleeps, all of these things need attention, especially as one continues to age.

<u>Grogginess in the Mornings</u>

If you wake up in the mornings feeling groggy, sluggish and in a sour mood, it is probably because of accumulated poisons and waste material that reside in you, not only in your colon but in the very tissues of your body. These poisons can be purged by eating living plant foods and watching the intake of harmful foods and drinks, and doing things that assist detoxification, such as colonics and enemas. Eating less food (a form of fasting) is also helpful.

Most people eat meat, cheese and their products thinking it does them good, because they are accustomed to believing that such foods are important to the body. However, they are doing the body much harm by eating them. Are meat, eggs, fish and cheese necessary for the body to heal? No, they are not.[305] For more information about how foods affect healing and vitality, see the book, *A Christian Diet*, listed in the Bibliography.

I used to suffer from various health issues, including constipation, stomachaches, headaches, hemorrhoids, psoriasis and other skin conditions, general fatigue, flatulence (excessive gas), broken sleeps and nightmares. In response to these "normal" conditions, entire industries have been created to produce prescription drugs to help people deal with them. Despite the availability of these

---

[305] See for example the books by Dr. Norman W. Walker, Dr. Ann Wigmore, Harvey Diamond and Arnold Ehret that are listed in the Bibliography.

drugs, I did my best to understand why, from a science of nutrition point of view, I was suffering from my conditions and what steps to I should take to correct them. I read all that I could about each condition. As it turned out, the conditions served as the catalyst I needed to change my diet to a whole plant food diet.

If you consume alcohol at night, it is important to eat alkalizing plant foods before retiring to bed to counteract the acidic blood chemistry caused by alcoholic beverages. It will give you better, sounder sleeps.

Exercise and Sleep

Exercise improves sleep. It helps us breathe deeper and flex the lungs. It strengthens the cardiovascular system. Exercise is known to improve mood and reduce feelings of depression and anxiety.

Toxins Removed During Sleep

A few results have appeared in brain research that indicate there is a connection between sleep and vitality.

Doctors at the Department of Human Health Sciences, Kyoto University Graduate School of Medicine in Japan, found that the quality of sleep a person gets directly affects a person's vitality. But this is only to be expected, since a lack of sleep adversely affects vitality.

Several years ago, Dr. Maiken Nedergaard, a professor of neurosurgery and co-director of the Center for Translational Neuromedicine at the University of Rochester Medical Center, discovered an important nervous system mechanism in the brain that prevents waste products from building up in the brain. She called it the "glymphatic system." The glymphatic system flushes any "debris" from the brain to the liver where it is eliminated.

According to the NIH (National Institutes of Health) Record of April 2015, Dr. Nedergaard reviewed a number of theories about what makes sleep a biological imperative, including its benefits to memory, the immune system and the preservation of human energy. She believes that sleep plays an important role in regulating the glymphatic system. Advanced imaging technology such as two-photon microscopy was used to examine the brains of live mice. The experiments compared the brains of mice that were awake, asleep and under anesthesia, to see if there was any difference in the way the glymphatic system worked to flush out the wastes from the brain. They found that during sleep, the glymphatic system was 10 times more active than when the mice were awake.

We always knew that sleep clears the brain and revitalizes us. Dr. Nedergaard's research indicates that there may be a connection between the preservation of human energy and the brain being cleansed of its waste products during sleep.

One never tires of sleep (!). There always seems to be a deficit of it that needs to be made up. While we may never succeed in creating a sleep pattern or environment that is entirely free of 3-AM wakeups or nightmares, we can reduce their frequency by eliminating some of their causes.

Want to feel your vitality returning after a good night's sleep? Be constipation-free.

Next Steps

For additional information, I encourage you to read the books listed in the Bibliography. They have much to offer the novice as well as the long-time student of foods and nutrition. We all like to eat, but it is only when we learn to eat foods that promote health, not destroy it, that our health flourishes. The books provide valuable information and inspiration that will help all seekers of health. They have been a constant source of encouragement to me on my health journey. Take the time to delve into them and you will be glad that you did.

About the Author

S. H. Shepherd, 74, has researched and studied the human health field for over 30 years. A scientist and engineer by training, his extensive knowledge of human health enabled him to cure himself and others of constipation. He has witnessed the decline of health in this country and the erosion of the quality of life that people suffer who have been stricken with this most troublesome and dangerous disease as well as various other health issues. He is firmly convinced that practically anyone can cure themselves of constipation and begin living the healthy and vibrant life that God wants them to live. The importance of telling others about the cure, as well as the many health hazards associated with commonly eaten foods, has been the incentive for writing this book.

The author has personally experienced many health issues that he was able to resolve as discussed in this book and in other books he has authored, which has given him a deep appreciation for the difficulties that others now or may have in the future.

Bibliography

1. T. Colin Campbell, The China Study, 2006.

2. Dr. Michael Greger, How Not To Die, 2015.

3. John Smith, Fruits and Farinacea- The Proper Food of Man, 2015.

4. Russell T. Trall, Scientific Basis of Vegetarianism, 1970.

5. Dr. Caldwell Esselstyn, Jr., Prevent and Reverse Heart Disease, 2007.

6. Jethro Kloss, Back to Eden, 2014.

7. Dr. Ann Wigmore, Be Your Own Doctor, 1982.

8. Dr. Ann Wigmore, Why You Do Not Have to Grow Old, 1985.

9. Dr. Ann Wigmore, The Sprouting Book, 1986.

11. Arnold Ehret, The Mucusless Diet Healing System, 2015.

11. Arnold Ehret, Physical Fitness Through a Superior Diet, Fasting, and Dietetics , 2018.

12. Arnold Ehret, Rational Fasting and Roads to Health and Happiness, 2002.

13. Arnold Ehret, The Cause and Cure of Human Illness, 2001.

14. Teresa Mitchell, My Road to Health, 1987.

15. Norman W. Walker, Colon Health, 2005.

16. Norman W. Walker, Become Younger, 1978.

17. Norman W. Walker, Fresh Vegetable and Fruit Juices, 1978.

18. Norman W. Walker, Diet and Salad Suggestions, 1985.

19. Norman W. Walker, Water Can Undermine Your Health, 1995.

20. Norman W. Walker, The Natural Way to Vibrant Health, 1972.

21. Norman W. Walker, <u>The Vegetarian Guide to Diet and Salad</u>, 1985.

22. Victoria Boutenko, <u>Green for Life</u>, 2005.

23. Victoria Boutenko, <u>12 Steps to Raw Foods</u>, 2005.

24. David Wolfe, <u>The Sunfood Diet Success System</u>, 2008.

25. David Wolfe, <u>Longevity Now: A Comprehensive Approach</u>, 2013.

26. David Wolfe, <u>Superfoods, the Food and Medicine of the Future</u>, 2009.

27. Dr. Joel Fuhrman, <u>Eat to Live: The Amazing Nutrient Rich Program for Fast and Sustained Weight Loss</u>, 2005.

28. Harvey Diamond, <u>Fit for Life Not Fat for Life</u>, 2003.

29. Harvey Diamond, <u>Living Without Pain</u>, 2007.

30. Dr. D. C. Jarvis, <u>Folk Medicine</u>, 1958.

31. D. C. Jarvis, <u>Arthritis & Folk Medicine</u>, 1960.

32. Robert O. Young and Shelly R. Young, <u>The pH Miracle</u>, 2010.

33. Paul C. and Patricia Bragg, <u>Apple Cider Vinegar, Miracle Health System</u>, 2008.

34. Paul C. and Patricia Bragg, <u>Miracle of Fasting</u>, 2005

35. Dr. Edward Howell, <u>Enzyme Nutrition</u>, 1985.

36. Paul C. and Patricia Bragg, Water, <u>The Shocking Truth That Can Save Your Life</u>, 2004.

37. Professor Spira, Spira Speaks, <u>Dialogs and Essays on The Mucusless Diet Healing System</u>, 2014.

38. Dr. Bernard Jensen, <u>Guide to Diet and Detoxification</u>, 2000.

39. Dr. Bernard Jensen, <u>The Healing Power of Chlorophyll</u>, 1973.

40. Fred S. Hirsch, <u>Internal Cleanliness</u>, 1987.

41. Tonya Zavasta, Beautiful on Raw Uncooked Creations, 2005.

42. Kristina Carrillo-Bucaram, The Fully Raw Diet, 2016.

43. Karyn Calabrese, Soak Your Nuts, 2011.

44. Herbert M. Shelton, Superior Nutrition, 1994.

45. Herbert M. Shelton, Fasting Can Save Your Life, 1978.

46. Herbert M. Shelton, Food Combining Made Easy, 1982.

47. Dr. Russel Blaylock, Excitotoxins, The Taste that Kills, 1997.

48. Joe Alexander, Blatant Raw Foodist Propaganda, 2005.

49. Horst Kornberger, Global Hive: Bee Crisis and Compassionate Ecology, 2012.

50. Annie Payson Call, Power Through Repose, 1905.

51. Steve Meyerowitz, Sprouts, The Miracle Food, 1997.

52. Dr. Henry Lindlahr, Philosophy of Natural Therapeutics, 1975.

53. Dan Georgakas, The Methuselah Factors, 1980.

54. Alexander Leaf, M.D., Youth in Old Age, 1975.

55. Andrew Weil, M.D., Healthy Aging, 2005.

56. Luigi Cornaro, Sure Methods of Attaining a Long and Healthful Life, 1660.

57. Luigi Cornaro, The Surest Method of Correcting an Infirm Constitution, 1660.

58. Luigi Cornaro, How to Live 100 Years, or Discourses on the Sober Life, 1660.

59. Dr. Johnny Lovewisdom, Dietetics Vitarianism, 2001.

60. Gabriel Cousens, M.D., Conscious Eating, 2000.

61. Jeffery M. Smith, Genetic Roulette, 2007.

62. F. Batmanghelidj, M.D, Your Body's Many Cries for Water, 2008.

63. Robert Morse, N.D., The Detox Miracle Sourcebook, 2004.

64. Arnold Paul De Vries, Therapeutic Fasting, 1958.

65. Dr. Kristine Nolfi, M.D., The Miracle of Living Foods, 1981.

66. T. Colin Campbell and Howard Jacobson, Whole: Rethinking the Science of Nutrition, 2014.

67. Wallace D. Wattles, Health Through New Thought and Fasting, 2007.

68. Francoise Wilhelmi de Toledo, MD, and Hubert Hohler, Therapeutic Fasting: The Buchinger Amplius Method, 2018.

69. Edward Hooker Dewey, M.D., The No-Breakfast Plan and the Fasting Cure. 1900.

70. Edward Hooker Dewey, M.D., The True Science of Living. 1894.

71. Upton Sinclair, The Fasting Cure, 1911.

72. Hereward Carrington, Vitality, Fasting and Nutrition, 1908.

73. Paavo O. Airola, N.D., There is a Cure for Arthritis, 1968.

74. Alfred Armand Montapert, The Supreme Philosophy of Man: The Laws of Life, 1977.

75. Edmond Bordeaux Szekely (Translator), The Essene Gospel of Peace, Book One, 1981.

76. Herbert M. Shelton, Health for the Millions, 1968.

77. O. L. M. Abramowski, Fruitarian Diet and Physical Rejuvenation, 1916.

78. Prof. Arnold Ehret's Mucusless Diet Healing System: Annotated, Revised, and Edited by Prof. Spira, 2015.

79. Sergei and Valya Boutenko, Eating Without Heating, 2002.

80. The Natural Hygiene Handbook, 1996.

81. Victoria Boutenko, Raw & Beyond, 2012.

82. The Complete Works of St. John of the Cross, Doctor of the Church, 2010:

83. G. Edmond Griffin, World Without Cancer, 2004.

84. Rich Anderson, Cleanse & Purify Thyself, 2000.

85. Elizabeth Lipski, Ph.D., CCN, Digestive Wellness, 2005.

86. Konstantin Monastyrsky, How to Prevent Nutritional Disorders and Premature Aging with Functional Nutrition, 1997.

87. Grady Ragsdale Jr.'s, Steve McQueen, the Final Chapter, 1983.

88. Margaret Hills, Treating Arthritis: The Drug-Free Way, 2007.

89. Arnold Ehret and Dr. Benedict Lust, Arnold Ehret's The Definite Cure of Chronic Constipation, 1922.

90. Stan Shepherd, Raw Veganism, 2018.

91. Stan Shepherd, Stop Sciatica and Spinal Stenosis, 2019.

92. Stan Shepherd, How to Heal Hemorrhoids: A Permanent Cure, 2020.

93. S. H. Shepherd, A Christian Diet, 2018.

94. S. H. Shepherd, The Cure for Arthritis, 2020.

95. S. H. Shepherd, Don't Take the Shots, 2022.

96. S. H. Shepherd, How to Cure High Blood Pressure, 2022.

97. Stan Shepherd, Raw Veganism, 2018.

Appendices

Appendix I, Berg's Tables

Appendix II, The Dirty Dozen and The Clean Fifteen

Appendix III, Bacteria in the Gut

Appendix I Berg's Tables

Ragmar Berg's Tables[306] list what foods are acid-binding and acid-forming. As explained in the chapter on The Causes of Disease, these terms are synonymous with mucus-binding and mucus-forming, respectively.

The larger the "plus" or "acid-binding" value, the more the mucus-binder or eliminator the food is. The larger the "minus" or "acid-forming" value, the more the mucus-producer the food is.

According to these tables, meat and grain products are the most acid-forming foods, whereas fruits and vegetables are most acid-binding foods. In other words, meat and grain products are the most mucus-producing foods, whereas fruits and vegetables are the most mucus-eliminating foods.

---

[306] Data taken from the tables published in Arnold Ehret's book, Mucusless Diet Healing System, and the tables available on the Web at the time of this writing.

The Only Cure for Constipation

Name of Food	Plus or Acid-Binding	Minus or Acid-Forming
Flesh		
Meat (Beef)		-38.61
Chicken		-24.32
Ham, Smoked		-6.95
Meat (Beef)		-38.61
Mutton		-20.30
Bacon		-9.90
Ox Tongue		-10.60
Pork		-12.47
Rabbit		-22.36
Veal		-22.95
Fish		
Herring, Salted		-17.35
Oysters	+10.25	
Salmon		-8.32
Shellfish		-19.52
Whitefish		-2.75
Eggs		
Eggs, Whole		-11.61
Eggs, White		-8.27
Eggs, Yolk		-51.83
Milk & Milk Products		
Butter, Cow		-4.33
Buttermilk	+1.31	
Cream	+2.66	
Lard		-4.33
Margarine		-7.31
Milk, Cow	+1.69	
Milk, Goat	+0.65	
Milk, Human	+2.25	
Milk, Sheep	+3.27	
Milk, Skim	+4.89	
Swiss Cheese		-17.49

The Only Cure for Constipation

Name of Food	Plus or Acid-Binding	Minus or Acid-Forming

Grains and Grain Products

Barley		-10.58
Black Bread		-8.54
Cakes (White Flour)		-12.31
Cornmeal		-5.37
Farina		-10.00
Graham Bread		-6.13
Macaroni		-5.11
Oat Flakes		-20.71
Oat Flour		-8.08
Oats		-10.58
Pumpernickel Bread	+4.28	
Quaker Oats		-17.65
Rice, Polished		-17.96
Rice, Unpolished		-3.18
Rye		-11.31
Rye Flour		-0.72
Wheat, Refined		-8.32
Wheat, Whole		-2.66
White Bread		-10.99
Zwieback		-10.41

Vegetables

Asparagus	+1.10	
Artichoke	+4.31	
Cabbages	+4.02	
Cauliflower	+3.09	
Chicory	+2.33	
Dandelion	+17.52	
Dill	+18.36	
Endives	+14.51	
Green Beans	+5.15	
Kohlrabi Root	+5.99	
Milk, Skim	+4.89	
Leeks	+11.00	
Lettuce, Head	+14.12	
Mushrooms	+1.80	

The Only Cure for Constipation

Name of Food	Plus or Acid-Binding	Minus or Acid-Forming
Red Cabbage	+2.20	
Red Onions	+1.09	
Rhubarb	+8.93	
Spinach	+28.01	
String Beans (Fresh)	+8.71	
Watercress	+4.98	

Root Vegetables

Black Radish, with Skin	+39.40	
Celery Roots	+11.31	
Horseradish	+3.06	
Red Beets	+11.33	
Sugar Beets	+9.37	
Sweet Potatoes	+10.31	
White Potatoes	+5.90	
White Turnips	+10.80	
Young Radish	+6.05	

Fruits

Apples	+1.38	
Apricots	+4.79	
Banana	+4.38	
Blackberries	+7.14	
Cherries	+2.57	
Cucumbers	+13.50	
Currants	+4.43	
Dates, Dried	+5.50	
Figs	+27.81	
Grapes	+7.15	
Lemons	+9.90	
Olives	+30.56	
Oranges	+9.61	
Peaches	+5.40	
Pears	+3.26	
Pineapple	+3.59	
Plums	+5.80	
Pomegranates	+4.15	

The Only Cure for Constipation

Name of Food	Plus or Acid-Binding	Minus or Acid-Forming
Prunes	+5.80	
Pumpkins	+0.28	
Raisins	+15.10	
Raspberries	+5.19	
Sour Cherries	+4.33	
Strawberries	+1.76	
Sweet Cherries	+2.66	
Tangerines	+11.77	
Tomatoes	+13.67	
Watermelon	+1.83	

Nuts

Acorns	+13.60	
Almonds		-2.19
Chestnuts		-9.62
Coconut	+4.09	
Hazelnuts		-2.08
Walnuts		-9.22

Legumes

Beans, dried		-9.70
Lentils		-17.80
Peanuts		-16.39
Peas		-3.41
Soy Beans	+26.58	

Drinks, Sweets

Cocoa		-4.79
Chocolate		-8.10
Tea leaves	+53.50	
Coffee	+5.60	

Appendix II The Dirty Dozen and The Clean Fifteen

Several years ago, the Environmental Working Group (EWG) published lists of fruits and vegetables known as the Dirty Dozen and the Clean Fifteen. These lists indicate foods with the most and least pesticide residues on them based on data compiled by the USDA. The lists are updated annually. They reflect pesticide residues found on foods after they were washed with water.

The Dirty Dozen

The foods highest on this list have the most pesticides on them.

1. Strawberries
2. Apples
3. Nectarines
4. Peaches
5. Celery
6. Grapes
7. Cherries
8. Spinach
9. Tomatoes
10. Sweet bell peppers
11. Cherry tomatoes
12. Cucumbers

According to EWG, buying organic for the twelve fruits and vegetables on this list can reduce our pesticide exposure by at least 90 percent!

The Only Cure for Constipation

The Clean Fifteen

The foods highest on this list have the least pesticides on them.

1. Avocados
2. Sweet corn
3. Pineapples
4. Cabbage
5. Sweet peas (frozen)
6. Onions
7. Asparagus
8. Mangoes
9. Papayas
10. Kiwi
11. Eggplant
12. Honeydew melon
13. Grapefruit
14. Cantaloupe
15. Cauliflower

There is no need to buy organic for the fruits and vegetables on this list, except for cabbage (number 4) and papayas (number 9). For cabbage, according to David Wolfe's book, *The Sunfood Diet Success System,* non-organic cabbage has large amounts of pesticides are used on it. Papayas are GMO foods and have pesticides.

Some types of produce are more prone to containing pesticides residues than others. Avocados, sweet corn and pineapples, for example, are not so prone because of their protective outer layer of skin. Not the same for strawberries and other berries.

Appendix III Bacteria in the Gut

The human body is host to trillions of microscopic organisms (microbes) that live in the skin, genitals, mouth, ears and sinuses, but the majority of them live in the "gut," a term which commonly means the stomach, but medically means the gastrointestinal (GI) tract, which was explained in the chapter on the Digestive System.

Called gut microbiota or gut microbiome, the bacteria in the gut perform many physiological functions. They help breakdown complex carbohydrates, proteins, and to a lesser extent fats that reach the intestines,[307] and protect the body against pathogenic microorganisms by regulating the response of the immune system, removing dead and dying cells, and fighting off invading microorganisms. [308] [309] [310] In fact, 70-80% of the cells of the immune system reside in the gut.[311]

Gut microbiota include the friendly (nonpathogenic) and the unfriendly (pathogenic) varieties, which, taken together, comprise a dynamic and complex population.

"A total of one hundred trillion bacteria live together in our digestive system, in either symbiotic or antagonistic relationships. That's ten times more intestinal bacteria than cells in our body. Their total weight is about four pounds – the size of the liver.

---

[307] https://microbiomejournal.biomedcentral.com/articles/10.1186/s40168-019-0704-8.
[308] https://bellalindemann.com/blog/side-effects-of-constipation#:~:text=Effects%20of%20constipation%20on%20FATIGUE&text=A%20lack%20of%20healthy%20flora,energy%20levels%20and%20cause%20fatigue.
[309] https://www.ncbi.nlm.nih.gov/pmc/articles/PMC3337124/.
[310] https://www.ncbi.nlm.nih.gov/pmc/articles/PMC7392086/.
[311] https://pubmed.ncbi.nlm.nih.gov/33803407/.

The Only Cure for Constipation

Eighty percent of the dry weight of our stools is composed of gut bacteria, and half of that is still alive." - Elizabeth Lipski, Ph.D., CCN, *Digestive Wellness*.

"The bacteria that live in our digestive tract are the largest organ of the body, even though they're not tied directly to the body through the blood supply." - Jeffrey Bland, Ph.D., Founder of Functional Medicine.

A healthy balance between the friendly and unfriendly bacteria in the gut must be maintained for health.[312] Many commonly eaten foods require long digestion times and consequently infrequent bowel movements; that is, many commonly eaten foods cause constipation and produce, in the fermenting wastes, an ideal breeding ground for the non-friendly parasites, including tapeworms, which can cause many health problems.

"Individuals with constipation often have significantly different gut bacteria composition than non-constipated, healthy people, with higher levels of methane [stinky gas] producing bacteria in their intestines, which slows intestinal transit time. A balanced microbiota, however, can reduce methane production, alter gut function, improve stool consistency and frequency, and help with constipation symptoms, including bloating, abdominal discomfort and pain."[313]

An imbalance of gut microbiota is medically called dysbiosis, which means the gain or loss of microbes that thrive in the

---

[312] https://www.webmd.com/digestive-disorders/ss/slideshow-how-gut-health-affects-whole-body#:~:text=In%20the%20gut%20microbiome.

[313] https://www.biogaia.com/health-areas/probiotic-gut-health/constipation/#:~:text=Individuals%20with%20constipation%20often%20have,which%20slows%20intestinal%20transit%20tim.

digestive system.[314][315]   An imbalance reduces bowel movement frequency, i.e., worsens a constipated condition, adversely affects immune system functioning, [316] and is responsible for many inflammatory diseases and infections that cause not only discomfort but can be life-threatening. [317] [318] [319] [320] [321]

Gut microbial composition and diversity (balance) are reduced, and therefore cause extended times between bowel movements by a nutrient deficient diet, eating too much sugar, and/or taking Ibuprofen and Aspirin, which are Nonsteroidal Anti-inflammatory Drugs (NSAIDs). Other factors that affect gut microbiota include tobacco use, excessive alcohol consumption, lack of exercise, and even chronic stress.[322] [323] [324]

Many people reach for Aspirin or some other drug that inhibits bacterial growth when something ails them. But drugs like antibiotics which are designed to wipe out the unfriendly or bad microbiota can also wipe out the good microbiota.

"Antibiotics may cause constipation in two ways. The first is by wreaking havoc with your gut bacteria and the second is by

---

[314] https://www.drelenaklimenko.com/constipation-relief-part-3-dysbiosis/.
[315] https://www.sciencedirect.com/topics/medicine-and-dentistry/dysbiosis#:~:text=2%20Dysbiosis.
[316] https://www.ncbi.nlm.nih.gov/pmc/articles/PMC3337124/.
[317] https://www.ncbi.nlm.nih.gov/pmc/articles/PMC6503315/.
[318] https://www.drelenaklimenko.com/constipation-relief-part-3-dysbiosis/.
[319] https://www.ncbi.nlm.nih.gov/pmc/articles/PMC5433529/.
[320] https://www.ncbi.nlm.nih.gov/pmc/articles/PMC5385025/.
[321] https://www.phlabs.com/taking-antibiotics-be-sure-to-protect-your-digestive-system.
[322] https://www.ncbi.nlm.nih.gov/pmc/articles/PMC5385025/.
[323] https://www.thegutmicrobiome.com/factors-that-influence-gut-microbiota/.
[324] https://www.hopkinsmedicine.org/health/conditions-and-diseases/constipation.

depleting your body of key minerals it needs for your gastrointestinal system to function at its best."[325]

Research has shown that it is best to encourage the growth of the beneficial bacteria to restore balance to the microbiome, rather than trying to get rid of the bad, or harmful, bacteria.[326] [327] [328] [329]

The healthy diversity of gut microbiota is best ensured when we eat vegetables and fruits.[330] [331]

The body is a most elaborately designed and intricate organism that must be held in balance in various ways for health to reign, and the most important way is by eating foods that keep the nonpathogenic gut bacteria in balance with the pathogenic bacteria, for when the balance is disrupted and the unfriendly bacteria thrive over their beneficial counterparts, disease reigns. In addition, many, if not most of the drugs used for constipation can adversely affect the balance of the bacteria.

Examples of the good bacteria are *Bifidobacterium and Lactobacillus.* Examples of the bad bacteria are *Clostridium and Staphylococcus.* You will often see the good bacteria listed on the labels of OTC (over-the-counter) probiotics that many people take to offset the damage done by eating a poor diet, and these supplements are discussed in more detail below.

---

[325] https://www.phlabs.com/taking-antibiotics-be-sure-to-protect-your-digestive-system.
[326] https://healthpath.com/gut-health/how-to-get-rid-of-bad-bacteria-in-the-gut/.
[327] https://pubmed.ncbi.nlm.nih.gov/28000678/
[328] https://www.ncbi.nlm.nih.gov/pmc/articles/PMC6320572/.
[329] https://www.ncbi.nlm.nih.gov/pmc/articles/PMC4303825/.
[330] https://www.ncbi.nlm.nih.gov/pmc/articles/PMC5385025/.
[331] https://www.fertile-gut.com/blogs/news/the-most-important-macronutrient-for-our-microbiome.

In addition to proper immune system functioning, researchers also believe that gut microbiota may be involved in the synthesis of larger molecules, such as amino acids, and are responsible for metabolic cross-organ signaling and insulin sensitivity.[332]

Since the balance of gut microbiota changes with age, some researchers believe that any imbalance accelerates the aging process.[333] If true, then promoting healthy gut microbiota by eating foods that are conducive to their health, and therefore also to a person's general health, could help people live longer.

Probiotics

Probiotics are commonly touted as miracle drugs when in fact they are substitutes for healthy foods. They are micro-organisms that are found in certain foods or come in supplements that augment or improve the good bacteria in the gut.[334] The World Health Organization (WHO) defines probiotics as "live microorganisms which, when administered in adequate amounts, confer a health benefit to the host."[335]

Probiotics are available in two broad forms, fermented foods and supplements. Fermented food products containing lactic acid bacteria, such as lactobacillus, include many pickled or soured foods, such as sauerkraut, sourdough bread, tempeh, miso, dairy products such as yogurt, kefir, buttermilk, and non-dairy products such as bee pollen, which have long been praised for their ability

---

[332] https://www.ncbi.nlm.nih.gov/pmc/articles/PMC5872693/.
[333] https://www.scientificamerican.com/article/gut-bacteria-change-as-you-get-older-and-may-accelerate-aging/#:
[334] https://www.mayoclinic.org/healthy-lifestyle/nutrition-and-healthy-eating/expert-answers/probiotics/faq-20058065.
[335] https://en.wikipedia.org/wiki/Probiotic.

to ease digestive difficulties, and are preferred health-wise over probiotic supplements.[336]

The supplements contain a wide array of different bacteria, two of the most common being Lactobacillus and Bifidobacterium. As promoted by the manufacturers and suppliers.

Both forms of probiotics give the gut microbiota food products they can thrive on. However, while probiotics may have some health benefits, one should beware of the many claims of probiotic manufacturers and suppliers that are designed to promote their sale, for evidence is lacking to substantiate them.

"Although numerous claimed benefits are marketed towards using consumer probiotic products such as reducing gastrointestinal discomfort, improving immune health, relieving constipation or avoiding the common cold, such claims are not supported by scientific evidence."[337]

It seems that probiotics are principally useful for people who eat nutrient deficient diets – such as the Standard American Diet – or have Crohn's disease or some other bowel disease, or who have poor health because of a sedentary lifestyle, all of which adversely affect gut microbiota balance. However, if you're eating a nutrient rich diet, such as a balanced diet of fresh fruits and vegetables, then you already have all the nutrients the body needs to feed your beneficial gut bacteria.[338] [339]

---

[336] Ibid.
[337] Ibid.
[338] https://www.novanthealth.org/healthy-headlines/do-you-need-probiotics.
[339] Ibid.

The Only Cure for Constipation

Probiotics should not be confused with *prebiotics*. Prebiotics are non-digestible food ingredients obtained from plant foods. Almost all plant foods have fibers that serve as fuel for the beneficial bacteria in the gut.[340] Unlike probiotics, which are basically bacteria that must feed on things to flourish, the prebiotics found in many whole plant foods, such as broccoli, cabbage, cauliflower, asparagus, avocados and blueberries, are excellent gut bacteria food.[341]

The immune system functions properly when the gut microbiota are fed foods that maintain microbiome balance. We maintain a healthy immune system by eating whole plant foods, including whole (raw) fruits and vegetables – properly combined if eaten together – and, at the same time, avoiding foods and their combinations that are known to be harmful to the body, such as those that cause stomachache, constipation, fermentation, gas and diarrhea – which are typical signals the body gives to warn us that something is wrong. Other signals may include anxiety and depression, precursors of a nervous breakdown, which in fact can be caused or partly caused by constipation.

Constipation caused by over-eating and improper food combinations is a major contributor to as mental unrest.

"The human nervous system is poisoned by impurities from the waste products of constipation which enter the bloodstream... Impurities in the blood supply to the brain makes normal functioning of that most important organ inefficient and befuddled." - Dr. Benedict Lust, *Overcoming Constipation Naturally*.

---

[340] https://www.gicare.com/gi-health-resources/prebiotics/.
[341] https://www.thehealthy.com/digestive-health/best-foods-and-recipes-for-gut-health/.

Index

A

Acidity, 57, 61, 98, 102-107, 129, 162, 165.

AGEs (advanced glycation end-products), 132, 182.

Alcohol, 61, 163, 203, 222..

Alternative medicine, 47, 79, 88.

Anus, 7, 12, 23, 25-27, 36-39, 111, 124-125.

Antioxidants, 89, 110, 127, 163, 172, 176-180, 192.

B

Bacteria, in gut, 221-227.

Berg's Tables, 105, 114, 126, 135, 193-194, 221-225.

Bowel, 4, 7, 20, 22-25, 35-36, 40-41, 51-52.

Bowel movement, 12, 14-15, 22-24, 36, 42, 46, 51-52, 56, 62, 77, 88, 91, 125-126, 148, 159, 209.

Bowel transit time, 26.

Brain disease, 5, 27, 61, 181-183, 187-188.

Bulk laxatives, 52- 54.

C

Caffeine, 53, 119, 163.

Cancer

    Colon or rectum (colorectal), 4, 18, 28, 30-34, 41, 44-45, 57, 162.

    Esophagus (esophageal), 28-30, 39.

    Liver, 21,23.

The Only Cure for Constipation

    Pancreas (pancreatic), 4, 28-30.

    Stomach (gastric), 4, 28-29.

Cholesterol, 135-136.

Coffee, see caffeine.

Colostomy, 144.

Colon, 4, 18, 27-28, 30-34, 35, 39, 41, 44-46, 51-52, 56-57, 66. 95, 97, 105, 108, 137, 144, 147-148, 157, 158, 162.

Colon hydrotherapy (irrigation), 158.

Colonoscopy, 31, 40, 45.

Cooked foods, dangers of, 87, 90-91, 112-113, 136-142, 147, 170, 183, 201.

Constipation, and acidity, 111-112, 114, 125-126, 170-171, 194.

Constipation, chronic, 22-27, 52, 148-149.

Corn, kernels, 125, 138, 163, 166-169, 194.

Cornmeal, 146, 169, 222.

COVID-19, 32, 95, 101-102, 119.

Crohn's disease, 20, 36.

D

Dehydration, 43-45, 52, 56, 69, 127.

Detoxification, 66, 85, 88-93, 100, 109, 114, 122-123, 158.

Diabetes, 18, 44-45, 98-99, 110, 119, 139, 163, 173, 181.

Diarrhea, 21, 23, 41-42, 54, 92, 162.

Diets

    American (traditional), 15, 20, 27, 32, 80, 87, 112-113, 137, 146, 150, 165, 172, 177, 185, 201-205, 207.

    Vegan, 109.

Raw vegan, 85, 109.

Digestion, 7-13, 71, 73, 76, 100, 111-113, 196-197, 199.

Digestion times, 9-11, 71, 75-76.

Diverticulitis and diverticulosis, 35-36.

Dysbiosis, 42-43.

E

Esophagus, 7, 28-29, 40.

Esophagogastroduodenoscopy (EGD), 40.

Enzymes, 7, 10, 83, 99, 113, 136, 138-143, 152-153, 176, 190-191, 197.

F

Fats, see Saturated fat.

Fatigue, 25, 34-36, 54-55, 66, 79, 91, 97, 140, 196.

Fasting, 68, 88-89, 103-104, 119, 142, 145, 151-152.

FDA (US Food and Drug Administration), 56, 63, 164.

Feces, 52, also see Stool.

Fiber foods, 33, 36, 38, 61, 137, 148, 161-169, 183, 195.

Food (GI tract) transit time, 10-12, 23, 26, 124, 169, 209.

Free radicals, 176-177, 179-180.

G

Gastrointestinal (GI) tract, 7, 10-13, 23, 25-26, 28, 33, 38, 123-124, 208.

GI bleeding, 39-40, 149.

Gluttony, 154-155.

Gut microbiota, 13, 22, 42-43, 120, 161, 165.

Gut microbial composition and diet, 13-14.

H

Hemorrhoids, 5, 25, 27, 37-39, 165, 146, 162, 169.

Hepatitis, 30.

Hydrochloric acid deficiency, 45-46.

I

Immune system, 29, 36, 39, 57, 92, 100, 110-113, 141, 169-170, 172, 185, 205, 221, 223, 225, 227.

Indigestion, 44, 57, 60, 64, 196.

Inorganic minerals, 187.

Irritable Bowel Syndrome (IBS), 10, 41.

K

Kidney disease, 5, 24, 44, 56, 59, 61, 95, 103, 110, 114, 145, 171.

L

Laxatives, 8, 47, 49, 51-57, 61-62, 95.

Leaky gut syndrome, 31, 35, 147.

Liver, 9-10, 14, 28, 30-31, 58-59, 61, 63, 67, 92, 105, 110.

M

Microbiome, 13, 57, 223.

Microbiota, see gut microbiota.

Milk, 19, 104, 110, 135, 161, 170, 186-189, 203-204, 221-222.

MSG, 71, 105, 179-180.

N

Nervous disorders, 5, 80, 87.

NSAIDs (Nonsteroidal Anti-inflammatory Drugs), 14, 42, 58-60, 147-149.

Nutritional deficiency, 45-46, 79, 105, 184-185, 187.

O

Obesity, 18, 45, 119, 129, 139, 153-156,163, 205.

Oils, Omega 6 oils, 9-10, 81, 106, 108, 125, 148, 195.

ORAC rating of foods, 178-180.

Osmotic laxatives, 52-55.

Overweight, see obesity.

P

Pancreas., 7, 10, 28-29, 141.

Patience, 87, 123.

Perforated colon, 45.

Peristalsis, 7, 69, 162-163.

Persistence, 206.

Prebiotics, 20.

Probiotics, 19-21.

R

Raw vegan diet, see Diets.

Rectum, 7, 23-24, 27-28, 31, 36, 39, 41, 51.

S

Saturated fat, 10, 119, 128, 145, 187.

Sigmoidoscopy, 40

Smoking, 78-79, 114, 223.

Starchy foods, dangers of, 74, 77, 88, 103-106, 108, 136-137, 143-147, 152, 169, 189, 194-195, 202.

Stimulant laxatives, 52-54.

Stomach, 4, 7-13, 24, 29, 39-40, 45-46, 57-58, 71-74, 75, 113-114, 148, 173, 196, 199.

Stool, 7, 12, 23-26, 29, 36, 38-39, 40, 43, 45, 52-53, 55-56, 62, 125, 161-162, 167, 209.

Stool softeners, 52-53, 55-56.

Stroke, 98, 109, 136, 182, 209.

T

Tobacco, 14, 222.

Toxicity, 89, 93, 101, 107-112, 145, 149, 155-156.

U

USDA (US Department of Agriculture), 164, 178, 187, 201, 203, 225.

Unsaturated fat, 184.

V

Vegan diet, see Diets.

W

Whole plant foods, 21, 67, 75, 84-85, 89-93, 98, 110, 120, 128-133, 141-142, 147, 152, 158, 164, 128, 171-172, 176-180, 181-199, 202-205.

Willpower, 206.

Wholistic approach, 26, 166.

Made in the USA
Monee, IL
26 March 2024